THE BOOK OF
LOVING SEX

THE BOOK OF
LOVING SEX

Nitya Lacroix

ULTIMATE
EDITIONS

First published in 1996 by Ultimate Editions
© 1996 Anness Publishing Limited

Ultimate Editions is an imprint of
Anness Publishing Limited
1 Boundary Row
London SE1 8HP

Distributed in Canada by Book Express
an imprint of Raincoast Books Distribution Ltd

ISBN 1 86035 079 8

A CIP catalogue record is available from the British Library

Publisher: Joanna Lorenz
Project editors: Casey Horton, Nicky Thompson
Design: Blackjacks
Special photography: Alistair Hughes
Additional photos: p94 Ron Sutherland/Science Photo Library;
p96 Jerry Wachter/Science Photo Library;
p97 Debbie Humphry © Photofusion
Hair and make-up: Bettina Graham

Printed in Singapore

Previously published as part of a larger compendium: *Love, Sex and Intimacy*

Contents

Chapter 1
Self-Awareness

Caring about your body and well-being is a major step in creating a strong sense of self-esteem. Developing a good relationship with yourself sets a solid foundation from which you can open yourself to a relationship with another person. The first place to begin is your body, because its health and vitality will give you the fitness and energy to enjoy your own life and to commit yourself with enthusiasm to another person. Simple steps can be taken which greatly enhance your life. A change to a healthy diet will give you the right balance of nutrition which will make you feel and look good. A regular programme of exercise, such as stretching, walking or aerobic work-outs will keep your muscles toned and your cardio-vascular system in good condition. Certain exercises, designed to deepen your breathing and unlock blocked emotional feelings, will bring you a greater sense of freedom and spontaneity. Then, taking good care of your skin and muscle tone by using self-massage techniques will help you to feel more relaxed and invigorated. Your self-awareness programme will make you feel positive about yourself and draw others to you.

Caring for Yourself

The gift of another person's love is a satisfying, fulfilling and nurturing force, but it is also important to gain that degree of caring and respect for yourself. We are not conditioned to love ourselves, but are encouraged to put our own well-being in second place in order to consider others. To create a secure sense of self-esteem involves a conscious drive towards self-awareness, and that is an ongoing process throughout our lives.

Building up your sense of self-worth will empower your life, and enable you to become less dependent on another person for your own feelings of personal value. This will sustain you in the times when you are on your own, and will also enrich any relationship you are involved in because you will have sufficient emotional resources to share.

You can start by planning a lifestyle that shows a real concern for the basics – a good diet, healthy exercise, and plenty of rest and relaxation. As well as enhancing your health and well-being, this will help you manage the tensions in your daily life so that stress becomes a power for good, for positive action and achievement, rather than a negative force that blocks and withholds your vital energy.

To have the confidence and enthusiasm you need to embark on a new relationship you have to feel good about yourself, and this means nurturing the essential you. This process of self-appreciation starts by ensuring you feel good internally and externally, so that your body is relaxed and full of energy and vitality, and your complexion is clear and glowing with life. Self-appreciation involves feeling good about your body so that you are content about yourself and life in general, as well as being very alive and spontaneous. It is also about preparing your physical self so that you are better able to fight disease and stay healthy, because ill health is a state of mind as well as body, and will dampen the enthusiasm and self-confidence you need to seek and sustain a loving relationship.

Ensuring you have adequate rest is an important part of this process. Never neglect your sleep routine because without sufficient rest and relaxation, your body is unable to replenish its resources, and you are unlikely to achieve the mental harmony you need to fulfil your potential.

Diet and Nutrition

Diet can often have the most direct and immediate effect on your well-being, and yet it is the one aspect of the average person's lifestyle that is most likely to be neglected. A healthy body must start with a healthy diet. That "you are what you eat" is an old adage – yet it is literally true, because the cells in your body are constantly being replaced by the molecules in your food. Food supplies the building blocks, in the form of amino acids and essential fatty acids, that repair and replenish your tissues, and ensure the normal functioning of the basic bodily processes. It also provides the vital energy you need to power you through the day and it will certainly add zest to your sexuality.

Mealtimes should be an important part of your daily activity. Instead of rushing your food, take time to sit down and relax as you eat. Turn your mealtimes into an occasion for mental relaxation as well as physical renewal. In this high-speed, high-pressure world it is tempting to forsake a good diet in favour of high-fat fast foods and sugar-rich snacks. This can only be a short-term solution and can have disastrous long-term consequences.

Vital Foods

◀ *A balanced diet that contains a wide range of foods, including plenty of fresh fruit and vegetables, will ensure you get all the vitamins and minerals you need for health and well-being.*

Eating too much of the wrong kinds of foods leads to a much higher risk of digestive disorders, heart disease, and certain types of cancer, as well as risking obesity and tooth decay. The body also needs adequate levels of essential nutrients, including vitamins and minerals, to stay healthy. Only by eating a balanced diet with a wide range of foods can you ensure that you are getting all the major nutritional components you need.

Highly processed foods invariably contain an excess of animal fats, and refined sugars, while much of the goodness, in the form of fibre and vitamins, is removed. These foods represent empty calories that add to your waistline but provide little else of benefit.

Physical well-being starts with a well-balanced diet. Normally, a person should aim to increase the percentage of complex carbohydrates, such as bread and potatoes, in the diet, and reduce the amount of refined sugars, such as cane sugar. Complex carbohydrates provide

Rest and Unwind
◀ Sleep relaxes the mind as well as the body by helping to uncoil the cares and tensions that have been building up throughout the day. It also refreshes and revitalizes you for the day ahead.

energy at a steady, sustainable rate, while simple sugars give a quick-acting energy surge that can make you edgy, hyperactive and irritable, and then leave you feeling drained and lethargic.

You should also try to cut down on saturated fat, obtained from meat and full-fat dairy products such as butter and cream, which clogs up the arteries and increases blood pressure levels. The ideal daily diet for a healthy adult should include:

❖ Up to eight glasses of pure water a day. This helps keep the kidneys functioning properly and flushes out the toxins and waste products that can build up in the body. You should also reduce your intake of stimulant drinks, such as tea, coffee and alcohol. These drinks can disrupt the body's fluid balance and over-stimulate the central nervous system, leading to insomnia, high blood pressure and raised heart rates, and aggravating stress disorders.

❖ Eat plenty of fresh fruit and vegetables, to provide the vitamins, minerals, and soluble and insoluble fibre you need.

❖ Have at least four servings a day of complex carbohydrates, such as bread (especially whole-wheat), pasta, rice, breakfast cereals, and potatoes.

❖ Include in your diet low-fat dairy foods, such as skimmed or semi-skimmed milk, yogurt, or

fromage frais. These provide the calcium and vitamins you need without significantly increasing your intake of saturated fats.

❖ Your daily intake of food should include two servings of protein foods such as chicken, fish, eggs, nuts, seeds, beans, peas and lentils. This gives the vital proteins needed to replace worn-out and damaged tissues. By including oily fish, such as herrings and mackerel, in your diet you will also be getting the essential fatty acids your body needs. A vegetarian diet can also be healthy and sustaining, but take care to ensure it contains the right balance of amino-acids.

Physical Fitness
It is important to take a well-balanced approach to your body. Without becoming neurotic about your size and weight, try to take an interest in your physical state because an enjoyable and invigorating fitness regime at a level you can sustain without undue stress can enhance your mental and physical well-being.

When you are unfit you tend to feel more lethargic and uninterested in the world and the people around you. If you are not in a current relationship, you may be less inclined to look for a partner. Low self-esteem about your own body may even transmit itself to others and be reflected in the way they regard you. Similarly, if you are in a partnership, your lack of vitality and enthusiasm could undermine your confidence and you may feel less inclined to put in the commitment required to sustain the relationship.

In addition, lovemaking is a physical activity and needs at least a minimum level of fitness. The fitter you are, the more likely it is that you will be in the mood for sex when your partner is feeling romantic, and the more enjoyment you will get out of lovemaking.

Regular exercise also provides major health benefits. It makes your heart, lungs and circulatory system work more efficiently, lowers cholesterol levels, and helps you to lose surplus fat and maintain your ideal weight once you have achieved it.

Releasing Vital Energy

In addition to the routines that help improve your general health and fitness, there are special exercises you can do to aid the release of muscular tensions within your body. Long-term tensions in the body, caused by emotional blocks and repressed feelings, can result in chronically tight muscles, and inhibit the free flow of vital energy – including sexual energy. This reduces your capacity to breathe deeply and prevents oxygen from reaching your inner core to replenish your vitality and nourish your cells and tissues.

Breath awareness, as described later in this book, and certain exercises can help relax and expand tense

Sideways Trunk Stretch

▲ This stretch exercise will help improve flexibility in your neck and body. Stand with your feet apart and take a deep breath. Bend sideways and breathe out. Hold the stretch for ten seconds. Repeat with the other side.

areas of the body, and allow for the release of pent-up emotional feelings. Chronic patterns of tension formed within the body are known as "muscular armour" and this needs to be released if the individual is to

gain greater emotional freedom and physical vitality.

The exercises shown here are based on Bioenergetic Therapy which is a system of bodywork devised by Alexander Lowen in the 1960s, and which has its roots in psychoanalysis. Lowen taught that a person's level of emotional stability is indicated by the degree of physical integration between one area of the body and another and the way he or she maintains contact with the earth through the feet and legs. This latter concept is termed "grounding". Grounded people "have their feet on the ground", literally as well as figuratively, and are rooted in the real world and in their physical reality, and so are better able to allow muscular-emotional release. Such individuals are better able to identify with the body and relate to their sexuality.

The following exercises – "the backward bow" and "the front drop" – may help you to increase your flexibility and sense of grounding by opening up areas of tension, and releasing stress, and so helping you gain access to your vital sexual energy. Try them to see if they are of benefit to you. Do

Limbering Up

Always start your exercise programme with a good limbering-up routine to stretch the stiffness out of the muscles and tendons. Be careful not to bounce or jerk as you do this or you may tear muscle fibres and damage joints.

Backward Bow

▶ *Stand with feet about 45cm/18in apart and toes turned in slightly. Make a fist with both hands and place them into your lower back. With knees well bent, and keeping your weight on the balls of your feet, arch your body backwards. Still keeping your weight forwards on your feet, breathe through the mouth and draw your breath deep down to your diaphragm. Hold this position for a minute to let the vibrations pass through your body.*

The Front Drop

◀ *Stand with your feet about 30cm/12in apart and your toes pointing in. Keeping your knees flexed, bend forward and touch the floor lightly with your fingers, without putting weight on your hands. Let your head hang down and keep your neck loose. Keep the weight of your body over the feet. Breathe easily through the mouth and take the breath a little deeper than usual. Slowly put the weight on the balls of the feet, without locking, or straightening the knees. Hold this position for a minute and then relax.*

both, one after the other, for about one minute each, and practise them every day, or three times a week, or whenever you feel the need to release tension. Always finish off with the front drop, even if you began with it, as this will release the tension from your lower back. (If you have a lower-back injury, these exercises should be used with caution or not undertaken until the condition has improved.)

Regarding the first exercise, the backward bow, Lowen points out in his book *The Betrayal of the Body* that the body arches like a bow to give itself impetus in various activities, such as when swinging an axe to cut wood, or serving a ball in a game of tennis. He states that this arc

movement is basic to sexual functioning and that any tension or disturbance which prevents the body from achieving the bow position, thus inhibiting a forward thrust, can diminish a person's ability to achieve sexual satisfaction.

This exercise draws attention to areas of tension within your body, particularly the diaphragm and abdomen, but because that area is put under stress by the position, it can begin to release its tension. Breathing should be through the mouth and deep enough to expand your belly. The energy release is felt as a trembling and shaking and, if this happens, simply allow it to vibrate through your body.

The second exercise, the front drop, has a dual purpose. By leaning forward the person is releasing tension blocks in the diaphragm that enable the breathing to become deeper and more revitalizing. In addition, because of the position of the feet and legs and the flexing in the knees, an individual is more aware of the contact with the ground and of tensions in the calf muscles and hamstrings.

As tension releases, this may be experienced as a tremor or tingling in the legs and possibly up towards the pelvis as stress areas are released and energy is able to flow freely. However, do not worry if you fail to experience this vibration at once.

Press-Ups

▶ *This strength exercise improves muscle tone in the shoulders and abdomen. Lie face down on the floor with hands at shoulder level, palms facing downwards, and elbows bent. Raise your body by straightening your elbows, while keeping your back straight. Hold for ten seconds, and then lower. Repeat five times.*

If you practise this exercise, daily or several times a week, you should begin to notice an effect.

Skin Care

As well as bringing about internal physical changes to enhance your self-esteem, a health and self-awareness routine can also take into account your outward appearance. Good grooming and a concern for your appearance is just as important for men as it is for women.

Helping to keep your skin clean and youthful looking does not need to involve expensive bills at a beauty parlour, or costly cosmetic preparations, as a simple daily regime is usually sufficient. A nutritious and balanced diet, of course, is the best way to have a healthy skin.

Skin care is mainly aimed at counteracting the harmful effects of the sun and wind, and preventing the pores becoming blocked by removing dirt and excess grease along with the outer layer of dead skin cells. You should avoid wearing heavy make-up and use a cleanser to remove all cosmetics before you go to bed.

Looking Good
▲ *Good grooming is just as important for men as it is for women. By taking some care over your appearance you encourage others to take an interest in you.*

Self-Discovery

Using creams and lotions to moisturize and revitalize your skin can make you feel sensual and help you to get in touch with your body. The insidious effect of advertising and its constant encouragement to achieve unrealistic perfection can often lead people, particularly women, to develop a negative body image. By massaging your own body with a good quality moisturizing cream or lotion to help nourish your skin, you can take the opportunity to explore your body so you learn to appreciate yourself, lose your negative feelings, and feel more positive, as well as caring for your skin at the same time.

Starting with your face, spread upwards and outwards from your nose, working the cream into your forehead and then sweeping out to the temples. Slide your fingers along the sides of the nose and out over your cheekbones, then use your fingertips to stroke upwards and outwards from your chin over the jaw and up to the ears. Finish this area by rubbing the cream into your neck, using an upward motion to tone the muscles.

Now use light sensuous touches of your fingers and palms to spread the

Air and Exercise
◄ *Aerobic exercise, such as jogging, will boost the heart and lungs and draw oxygen into the tissues to improve your health, well-being and mental alertness.*

cream over your body. Working outwards from your heart, spread the cream across your chest, using an upward motion on your breasts, and then rub it over your shoulders and down your arms. Work from your lower breastbone over your belly and down your legs to your feet. Take time to rub the cream in well, particularly into the top and undersides of the feet, to squeeze out the muscular knots and tensions that can accumulate here.

Alternatively, using a similar technique, spread a rich massage oil over your body. A man should pay particular attention to the muscles around the shoulders and arms and in the legs, stroking and kneading the flesh with the fingertips to loosen and invigorate the muscle fibres.

To enhance the feeling of relaxation and contentment, blend one or more aromatherapy oils into your massage lotion. Lavender is a safe and attractive oil for relaxation and harmony which can also ease tired, stiff, or aching muscles, but there are many more you can choose.

By using these soothing caresses on your skin, you will begin to know and love your body, as well as nurturing your skin with the lotion to leave it soft and glowing. As you stroke over your skin, let your hands relax so they are able to slide smoothly and sculpt over your body's contours.

Self-Massage

A regular self-massage programme makes you look and feel more relaxed, as well as stimulating the circulation and enlivening your skin so that you can become more sensually responsive. It can help you develop an awareness of your outer self, as well as dispelling negative thoughts, and improving your body image.

Start off by massaging the head, using tiny circular movements, as if shampooing your hair, and feel the scalp move under your fingers. Now massage the temples, using two fingers of each hand in a circular motion to relieve mental tension, and then work on the fleshy areas of your

Care and Attention

◀ *Apply a good quality moisturizing cream to nourish your skin, and explore your face and body at the same time, so you can learn to appreciate yourself as you care for your complexion.*

cheeks, using the flats of your fingers in large circular movements.

The next stage is to follow an invigorating sequence of massage strokes to refresh and revitalize your skin and muscles. Start with the face, and use the tips of your fingers to tap all over the facial muscles, jaw-line, forehead, temples and cheeks. Next, work on the shoulders and neck. Make a loose fist and use the flat surface of the fingers to pummel the muscles gently. Use the same technique to pummel the arms and down to the backs of the hands. Now do the same thing on the inside of the hands and arms, before using alter-

nate strokes to pound the ribcage vigorously. Finally, use a hacking motion with the side of the hands on the legs and feet to tone up the muscles and boost the circulation.

A very invigorating massage can be obtained by using a skin brush. This device, which is available from health shops, is used dry and stroked over the skin. It removes the outer layer of cells and allows the underlying cells to regenerate themselves. It revitalizes and tones the skin and enhances the body's ability to eliminate toxins, as well as leaving the skin soft and smooth to the touch.

Starting at your feet, work up your legs and then your arms, and over your body towards your heart, following the direction of your circulation. Follow it up with a shower to wash off any remaining dead skin cells. You can do this several times a week to leave your skin glowing with health and vigour, and silky soft to the touch.

Massage the Muscles

▼ *Spread a massage oil over your body, working it into the muscles of the shoulders, arms, and legs. Knead the flesh with the fingertips to loosen and relax the muscle fibres.*

Pummel the Tissues

▼ *By making your hands into a loose fist you can gently pummel the body to release tension in the tissues and boost the blood circulation, leaving you feeling restored and invigorated.*

Brush Your Skin

▼ *Use a skin brush to remove the dead outer layer of skin cells. It will revitalize and refresh the skin and also leave your body tingling and glowing with health and vitality.*

Chapter 2

The Sexual Body

Our sexual body is a miraculous part of our psychosomatic reality, yet generally we know little about how it develops and functions. In this chapter, we discuss how our sexual organs mature through adolescence to adulthood and begin to unravel the mysterious differences between the male and female reproductive systems. To understand our sexuality fully, we must first make the effort to get to know the geography of our sexual systems, and learn about their physical processes, strengths and weaknesses. Then we can go on a voyage of discovery in search of the body's secret pleasure zones – a journey which can bring us sexual happiness.

The Woman's Body

Throughout history, the female body has been regarded as a potent symbol of fertility and sexuality – both mystifying and feared. In the past, women have sometimes felt that their bodies do not even belong to them because they are viewed as objects by society at large. Now, more than ever, women want to feel they are in charge of their own bodies. Learning to know your body, and understanding how it functions, is an important step in this process. This section provides basic information on the sexual and reproductive nature of a woman's body, the changes that occur at puberty, and some of the other physical and psychological processes that take place on the journey from girlhood to womanhood.

Woman and Art

▶ *The beautiful symmetry of a woman's body, its rounded contours and sensual shape, has inspired great paintings, songs, poetry, and works of literature.*

The Breasts

A woman's breasts are a symbol of her femininity, for their spherical softness is very sensual, regardless of size. The breasts are sexually responsive to tactile stimulation and they will swell slightly during sexual arousal. The nipple and the areola, the dark pigmented skin which surrounds the nipple, are also highly sensitive to touch. The nipple is made up of erectile tissue and enlarges when stimulated. While a woman's breasts are often regarded as sexual organs, their primary function is to produce milk to nourish a baby. Each breast is made up of around 20 lobes, containing numerous milk-producing glands, which are surrounded by fatty tissue. Tiny tubes – called the lactiferous ducts – carry the milk to small openings in the nipple. The breasts contain no muscles, but strands of ligament weave in between the tissues to give them their shape and support. The size of the breasts varies greatly from woman to woman, but bears no relation to the quantity of milk they can produce.

The Vulva

Vulva means visible and refers to the external female genitalia, or that which can be seen. This mainly consists of the mons, the labia majora and minora (the outer and inner "lips"), and the clitoris.

Diagram labels: clitoral hood, mons pubis, labia majora, labia minora, vestibule, clitoris, urethra, vagina, perineum, anus

Breast Size

Breast shape and size varies greatly between women. The way a woman with a 34 inch bust (the average breast size) feels about her breasts may partly depend on the era and culture she is born in. Fashions in what is considered an attractive breast size change constantly, from the buxom and curvaceous style favoured by Hollywood in the 1950s to the small and boyish, almost androgynous shape of many of today's top models.

It is important for a woman to love and accept her body – particularly the shape of her breasts – the way it is, for it is an expression of her own unique femininity. If the breasts are large and causing discomfort it will help to wear a good support bra. Small breasts cannot be enlarged directly by exercise as they do not contain muscle, but good posture (a lengthened spine, and straightened shoulders) can lift the ribcage to give the breasts a more pronounced shape. Likewise, you can develop the underlying pectoral muscles, which may help increase the lift and support the weight. A difference in size between the left and right breast is very common.

Breast Skincare

◀ *Taking care of the thin skin which covers the breasts can help to prevent stretch marks. Rub moisturizing cream on and around the breasts to keep the skin soft and smooth.*

Variety of Shapes

▼ *Nipple shapes and sizes are also very varied. Some nipples are naturally inverted – the nipple is pulled inwards and hidden behind a fold in the skin. In most cases, inverted nipples should not prevent successful breastfeeding. If, however, a nipple suddenly becomes inverted during adulthood, it is important to consult a doctor immediately, as this may indicate breast cancer.*

Mons Pubis

The mons, or mons pubis, is also rather romantically known as the mons veneris, or Mount of Venus. It is the soft mound of fatty tissue, covered by skin and pubic hair, which protects the pubic bone from friction during intercourse. Its rich supply of nerve endings makes it very sexually responsive to tactile stimulation.

Pubic Hair

The pubic hair which covers the mons grows in a triangular shape and sometimes spreads down to the thighs. It is darker and coarser than head hair. It can be thick or sparse, and these differences can be particularly marked between races. It also thins with age. Cultural influences usually dictate whether women shave or wax their pubic hair, or let it grow. Pubic hair is one of the first signs of sexual development.

Labia Majora (Outer Lips)

The word labia means lips. The labia majora are the two outer fleshy folds of skin and fatty tissue. When a woman is sexually excited, the lips become engorged with blood and swell. They are partly covered with pubic hair.

Labia Minora (Inner Lips)

The labia minora are two fleshy folds of skin which are mostly covered by the labia majora, although they may protrude. The inner labia, in turn, cover the urethra, or urinary opening, and the vagina. There are many variations among women in the shape, size and colour of the labia minora. The labia meet to form a hood over the head of the clitoris and extend to just below the vaginal opening. They are richly supplied with nerve endings. Unlike the outer lips, they are not covered with pubic hair. The cleft between the labia minora is known as the vestibule. Ducts from Bartholin's glands, which secrete a lubricant when a woman is sexually excited, open into the vestibule. This lubricant reduces skin friction and so enables easier penetration of the vagina during intercourse.

Clitoris

The clitoris is located where the inner labia meet. In Greek folklore, the sunflower, Kleite, grew and opened when stimulated by the sun, an apt analogy for this most sexually sensitive part of a woman's body. The clitoris is made of erectile tissue similar to that of the glans of the penis, and is as richly supplied with nerve endings as the penis, though concentrated within a much smaller area. The clitoris can measure 2–5cm/ ³/₄–2in, but appears smaller as only the top is visible. It is partly covered

Self-Discovery

Many women feel very shy about their genital area, and may never have seen it properly for themselves. In this respect, men are luckier, as they can not only see their own genitals easily, but their partner's too. To help you get to know, love and understand your body better, try this exercise to examine and explore your vulva and vagina.

Using a hand mirror will enable you to see this hidden part of yourself. Find a comfortable position, either squatting or lying on your back propped up on pillows, and angle the mirror to give yourself a full view of your external genitalia. As you look, explore each part with your hands and fingers. Notice the shape and colour of your labia, and part the outer lips to get a closer look at the inner, fleshy folds. Seek out your clitoris, and gently stroke it with a finger. Then explore the outer entrance to your vagina, allowing a finger to penetrate gently in order to feel the soft, mucous membranes of its inner wall.

by the labia minora and fills with blood when a woman is sexually excited. The clitoris has no obvious purpose other than to give pleasure to a woman, and with skilful manipulation during masturbation or love-making, it is instrumental to her achieving an orgasm.

Hymen

The hymen is a thin fold of tissue that partly covers the entrance to the vagina. Undamaged, it has a small central opening which allows the outflow of menstrual blood. The hymen is easily torn or stretched during strenuous activity in childhood, by the insertion of tampons, or, in later years, by sexual intercourse. Once broken, the ragged edges of the hymen tissue ring the vaginal opening. Contrary to former belief, a broken hymen does not necessarily mean that a woman is not a virgin.

Vagina

The vagina (which means sheath) is a channel measuring 7–10cm/2³⁄4–4in leading from the vulva to the uterus. The entrance to the vagina is located just below the urethra, or urinary opening. The muscular walls of the vagina are deeply folded so that it can expand during intercourse or childbirth. They are also richly supplied with blood vessels, which become engorged with blood during sexual arousal. The walls are covered with a mucous membrane which secretes a fluid that helps lubricate the vagina, especially during intercourse. These secretions are slightly acidic, which helps to keep harmful organisms in check. The vagina also acts as an outlet for the flow of menstrual blood.

Cervix

The cervix is the neck of the uterus and is located at the top of the vagina. It is a narrow, cylindrical structure, made of tough tissue and muscle, and is approximately 2.5cm/1in long. In the centre of the cervix is the os, a small opening which enables sperm to pass into the uterus and allows menstrual blood to flow out. It remains firmly closed during pregnancy, while the rest of the uterus expands to accommodate the foetus. During the final stages of labour, in response to contractions of the uterus, the cervix dilates to allow the baby to pass through into the birth canal. A special form of mucus is secreted by glands in the cervix. The consistency of the mucus changes throughout the menstrual cycle, becoming profuse, slippery and stretchy, clear or slightly cloudy around the time of ovulation, when it is called fertile mucus, and sticky, white or even absent afterwards. Fertile mucus plays an important role in reproduction by aiding the passage and survival of sperm.

Uterus

The uterus, or womb, is a muscular organ, roughly the shape of an upside-down pear, located above and behind the bladder. It is 7.5–10cm/3–4in long, on average, and weighs 60–90g/2–3oz. During the menstrual cycle, the lining of the uterus (the endometrium) increases in thickness as it prepares to receive and nourish a fertilized egg. If this does not happen, the lining breaks down and is shed during menstruation. During pregnancy the uterus expands and becomes more muscular to contain the developing baby. These muscles also produce powerful contractions during labour to expel the baby.

Fallopian Tubes

The Fallopian tubes are about 7.5cm/3in long and attached at either side to the upper end of the uterus, with an opening no wider than the eye of a needle. The other end of each tube, the ampulla, is funnel-shaped and has finger-like frills called fimbriae. When an egg is released from the ovary, these fimbriae waft it into a Fallopian tube. The egg is then carried along the tube and into the uterus by the action of hair-like projections called cilia and by contractions of the tube walls. Fertilization usually occurs within a Fallopian tube. Occasionally, a fertilized egg may implant in the wall of a Fallopian tube and continue to develop, resulting in an ectopic pregnancy – a potentially life-threatening condition.

Ovaries

The ovaries are almond-shaped organs about 3cm/1¼in long. They produce the eggs, or ova, which, when fertilized by sperm, develop into a human life. The ovaries are located just behind and to either side of the uterus and lie close to the funnel-shaped ends of the Fallopian tubes. Around 600,000 immature eggs are present at the start of a woman's fertile life, although only

around 400 will develop into mature eggs. The eggs develop in special sacs, called follicles. During each menstrual cycle one egg only usually bursts out of its follicle and is collected by the fimbriae of the nearest Fallopian tube. The ovaries also produce two hormones, oestrogen, mainly responsible for female sexual development, and progesterone which causes the lining of the uterus to thicken, ready to receive a fertilized egg. If fertilized, the egg will then embed itself in the lining, where it will develop into a foetus.

Female Sexual Development

Puberty in females starts at around the age of ten, triggered by an upsurge in the level of sex hormones secreted into the bloodstream, and can take up to five years to complete. The start and rate of development of a girl's sexual maturity differs from one individual to another, but may be

influenced by hereditary factors, nutrition and health. The improvement in diet and living standards in industrialized nations is thought mainly responsible for the earlier onset of the first menstrual cycle in girls today.

The initial changes in puberty, between the ages of ten and 12, are triggered by chemical and nerve signals from a region in the brain called the hypothalamus. These signals cause the pituitary gland, just below the brain, to release hormones called gonadotrophins. These, in turn, instruct the ovaries to start releasing the hormones oestrogen and progesterone. The various hormonal changes at this time bring about a sudden spurt in growth, including increased height and muscle weight, changes in the distribution of fat around the body, and the development of the reproductive organs.

The first changes may be the budding of the breasts, one often earlier than the other, and the darkening of the pigment of the areolae. This is usually followed by the appearance of pubic hair, and then underarm hair. The uterus, Fallopian tubes and ovaries start to mature, the vagina enlarges, and the labia begin to swell. There may also be an increase in vaginal secretions, and the oil and sweat glands become highly active, often leading to acne and pimples.

The characteristic female shape now begins to develop, as the pelvis widens and fat deposits are laid down under the skin of the breasts, buttocks, hips and thighs. The first menstrual period, the menarche, occurs on average between the ages of 12 and 13 years, but usually not

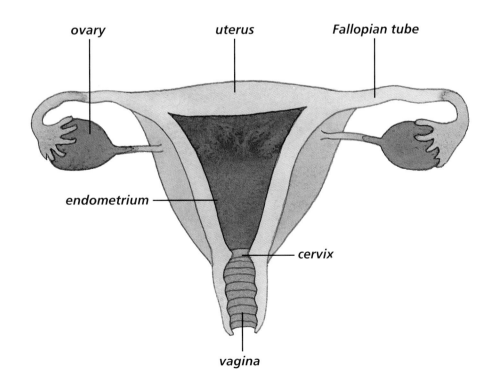

ovary   uterus   Fallopian tube

endometrium

cervix

vagina

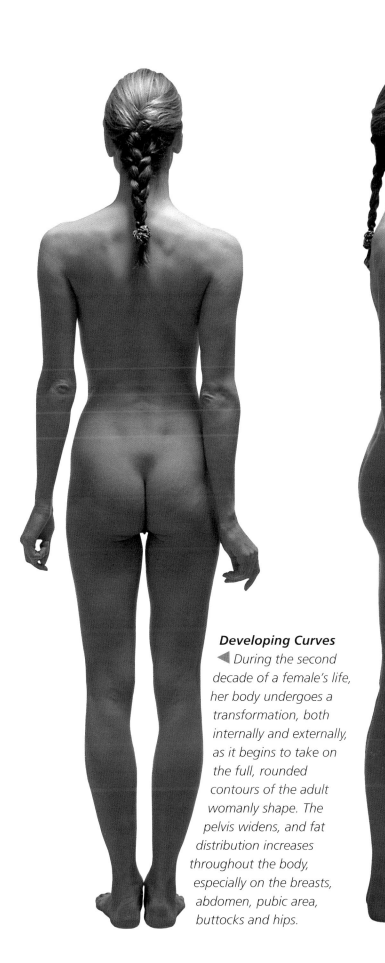

until at least a year after the secondary sexual characteristics have begun to develop. The start of regular periods marks the completion of puberty.

From Girl to Woman

An adolescent girl may welcome the dramatic changes in her body as evidence that she is entering womanhood. Equally, she may be distressed or alarmed by them, feeling that her body is out of control, or being reluctant to relinquish her childhood so soon. She is likely to go through intense mood swings, partly due to hormonal fluctuations, but also because she must adapt psychologically as well as physically to her new identity.

She is no longer a little girl and, in various ways, she may demand that her changing identity is recognized by her family. A young teenage girl may need to assert her developing womanhood, separating herself temporarily from the close bond she had previously shared with her mother. Her relationship with her father may alter as they both try to find a new way of acknowledging and adjusting to her developing sexuality. At this point, a father may stop showing his normal displays of physical affection, unsure of exactly how to relate to his daughter.

Developing Curves

◀ During the second decade of a female's life, her body undergoes a transformation, both internally and externally, as it begins to take on the full, rounded contours of the adult womanly shape. The pelvis widens, and fat distribution increases throughout the body, especially on the breasts, abdomen, pubic area, buttocks and hips.

Arrival of Womanhood

◀ In the later stages of puberty, a female's menstrual cycle usually becomes more regular, on average settling at between 26 and 32 days' duration. Her breasts develop to their adult size, her pubic hair becomes thicker, and underarm hair appears. By now, her voice may have become slightly deeper. A female's growth in height slows down soon after puberty.

A Need to Bond
▼ *On the whole, women of all ages consider intimacy, love and emotional bonding to be an important part of forming a sexual relationship*

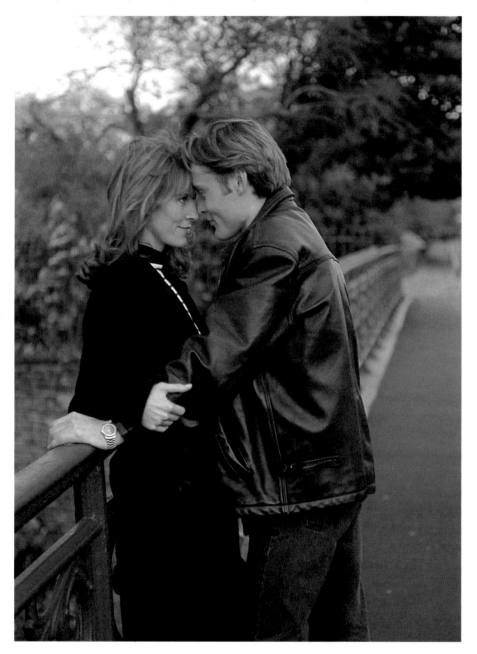

In spite of these difficulties, the adolescent girl will need a great deal of emotional support from her parents, even though she appears to challenge them on every issue.

Sex Education
It is important that a girl is fully informed about the physical changes her body will undergo during puberty, and has adequate knowledge about menstruation, and related hygiene matters, before her periods begin.

It is not always easy for parents to discuss sexual issues with their children although, nowadays, families do tend to be more open about such topics. If the mother, or guiding parent, feels unable to discuss these subjects with the daughter (girls may also find it embarrassing to discuss sexual matters with their parents), it is important to find someone the girl can trust and who will answer her questions, or provide her with suitable books from which she can gather accurate information. Informed sex education is not a green light for promiscuity.

A teenage girl will benefit from knowing that during adolescence she is likely to feel attracted to boys, and even experiment in sexual play with them, and that sometimes her emotions and sexual feelings will be overwhelming. She needs to understand the importance of defining the boundaries of her sexual behaviour so that she is able to resist male or peer group pressure to engage in any sexual activity for which she does not feel ready. By discussing these issues with an understanding adult, she will be better equipped to take control of her body and emotions.

Studies show that adequate sex education for young people (males and females) about contraception, sexually transmitted diseases, and the complexities of emotional and sexual feelings in relationships, can help reduce cases of premature sexual intercourse and of teenage pregnancies.

Sexual Experience
Young women do masturbate, for sexual release and to explore their bodily responses, although slightly less often than males of the same age. According to research, the average age for the loss of virginity in young women in the United States and Great Britain is between 16 and 18. There are still many young women who, for religious, romantic or moral reasons,

or through fear of pregnancy, or sexually transmitted disease, prefer to remain virgins until they meet a man with whom they can develop a committed relationship. However, in most western cultures there is no longer the same pressure on females to remain virgins until their wedding night, and many young women will have had several sexual partners by the time they reach their twenties.

These days, women expect to compete equally with their male colleagues in the academic and work environment, and for most women marriage and children are no longer seen as their only goals. The wider availability of contraception has given women greater freedom in all areas of their lives.

Increasingly, women are choosing to live with a partner before marriage, and to delay starting a family until established in a career. It

A Growing Capacity for Sexual Arousal

▲ *As a woman's sexual experience increases, so does her orgasmic capacity. When she is fully relaxed in her body, and is aroused lovingly by a sensitive and knowledgeable partner, her sexual pleasure is almost boundless.*

is not unusual for women to wait until their thirties before having their first baby – and some are now leaving it until their forties to start a family – and most expect to return to work within a few months or years after giving birth.

Women's Sexual Peak

A woman's capacity to achieve an orgasm appears to increase with age and sexual experience. Women tend to reach their sexual peak during their thirties and can continue at this level for many years. In part, this may be because as a woman gets older and becomes more confident and relaxed in her sexuality, she is better attuned to what will bring her

sexual satisfaction during lovemaking. Younger women may be more preoccupied with trying to please their partners during intercourse, while, in general, women are more sexually responsive when they are involved in a secure, intimate and loving relationship.

Although women are becoming more sexually assertive and better able to initiate relationships with the opposite sex, they still suffer from society's double standards over the morality of multiple sexual experience. Whereas a man is expected to "sow his wild oats" as evidence of his virility, a woman can still be regarded as promiscuous if she has had several sexual partners.

The Man's Body

Men are conditioned to be less self-conscious about their bodies than women, but nevertheless, men still have many concerns about their physical selves which they are often unable to express verbally. Gender conditioning varies greatly between cultures but, in general, men are usually expected to sublimate their more vulnerable, gentle, and sensitive feelings and to place more emphasis on the development of physical prowess. Yet a man's reproductive system is complex and miraculous, involving him on both a physical and emotional level. This section will aim to explain the form and function of the male sex organs, and will look at a man's sexual and psychological adventure through life.

The Classic Male Image

◀ The masculine form traditionally symbolizes strength and virility, and this depiction of the athletic manly physique has been a popular theme in classic sculpture and art. The more emotional and sensual aspects of the male psyche have received far less acknowledgement.

Learn About Each Other

▲ Men and women can benefit enormously from learning about each other's sexual anatomy. It is important to understand the differences between the two – and also the similarities.

The Scrotum

The scrotum is the pouch which contains and supports the testicles, hanging down externally below the pubic bone and behind the penis. It is made up of a layer of contractile muscle covered by a pouch of thin, loose skin. While the scrotum looks like one sac, it is actually divided into two compartments, each housing one testicle. The external location of the scrotum helps to keep the sperm at their optimum temperature of two or three degrees below normal body heat. If the outside temperature drops, the scrotum is drawn closer to the warmth of the body so that the testicles are not allowed to get too cool.

Testicles (Testes)

The testicles, or testes, are the male reproductive organs. Each testicle is suspended from a thick fibrous structure called the spermatic cord. During the early stages of foetal development the testicles are located high within the abdomen, but they slowly descend until at birth they have arrived at their final position. They are composed of two types of cells – one type makes sperm, while the other produces the male sex hormone testosterone. Each testicle contains an intricate and convoluted network of coiled tubes, the seminiferous tubules, in which the sperm cells develop. Sperm then pass into a larger coiled tube, the epididymis, where they are stored until they mature.

Vas Deferens (Seminal duct)

Mature sperm are stored in the vas deferens, an elongated tube contained within each spermatic cord, and are pushed towards the urethra by muscular contractions. During a

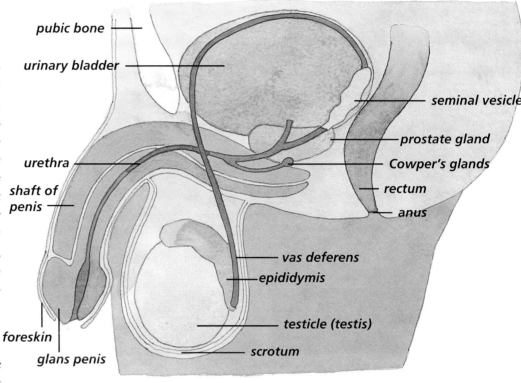

vasectomy, the male form of sterilization, each vas deferens is cut and tied to prevent sperm from leaving the testicles. After sterilization, although sperm continue to be produced, they are reabsorbed into the body. The operation does not prevent the ejaculation of sperm-free seminal fluid.

The Prostate Gland

The prostate gland, which is about the size of a chestnut, is situated in front of the rectum and just below the bladder. It secretes some of the seminal fluid, or ejaculate, which helps transport the sperm, and also produces a lubricant to keeps the lining of the urethra moist. The prostate gland can produce highly erotic sensations if directly stimulated by a partner's lubricated finger inserted into the anus, which is why it is sometimes said to be the male equivalent of the female's G-spot.

Seminal Vesicles

The seminal vesicles are two long sac-like organs located near the prostate gland at the junction of the two vasa deferentia and the urethra. They secrete about 60 per cent of the seminal fluid, which passes through the prostate gland and into the urethra via the ejaculatory ducts. The secretions from the seminal vesicles are high in sugars which will help provide the nourishment the sperm need on their long journey to fertilize the egg.

Cowper's Glands

The Cowper's glands are two pea-sized glands situated below the prostate and on each side of the bulbous portion of the urethra. Their ducts exude a clear, alkaline fluid into the urethra which helps protect the sperm by neutralizing the acidic environment of the urethra.

25

Penile Erection

▼ *A full penile erection, commonly known as a "hard-on", is due to blood being pumped into the erectile tissues at a much faster rate than it can escape. This causes the tissues to swell and the penis to enlarge.*

Urethra

The urethra is the channel through which both urine and semen pass out of the body. It originates at the bladder and passes through the prostate gland and the shaft of the penis before terminating at the external urethral opening, situated in the glans, or head of the penis. The male urethra is up to 20cm/8in in length – much longer than the female urethra. To prevent urine escaping with the semen, a ring of muscle closes off the bladder prior to ejaculation.

Penis

Most men would regard the penis as the most important part of their sexual anatomy and it is certainly their most erotically sensitive area. The penis consists of erectile and fibrous tissue and involuntary muscle, with a rich supply of nerves and blood vessels, surrounded by skin. The spongy erectile tissue of the

penis is made up of three cylindrical compartments. These are the two corpora cavernosa and the corpus spongiosum, which surrounds the urethra. During sexual arousal, these cylinders fill with blood, causing the penis to grow erect.

The head of the penis is called the glans. The external urethral opening, through which semen is ejaculated, is in the centre of the glans. In uncircumcised men, the head of a flaccid penis is normally covered with a fold of loose skin called the foreskin, or prepuce. During erection the foreskin is stretched back to expose the glans, and this exposure is further increased by friction during coitus. The glans is very well served with nerve endings, and is the most erotically sensitive part of the man's penis. Where the skin folds back just below the under-ridge of the glans is an area called the frenulum. This is also very responsive to sexual stimulation.

A full erection of the penis can sometimes occur within seconds of sexual stimulation, although sexual arousal does not automatically lead to an erection. This can sometimes be a cause of great anxiety for men who are worried about their sexual performance.

Facts About Sperm

Sperm take about ten weeks to develop inside the testicles. Up to 30 billion sperm are produced each month and 50–100 million sperm per millilitre are present during a single ejaculation, which produces about one teaspoon of semen. In each ejaculation up to 40 per cent of sperm may be deformed or inactive. Sperm that are not ejaculated are reabsorbed into the body. Each microscopic-sized sperm has an oval head, a tubular mid-section, and a whip-like tail. The head contains 23 chromosomes – half the normal

Penis Sizes

Most men have worried about the size, shape and performance of their penis, at one time or another. This is hardly surprising since men are constantly being subjected to the concept of the mythical penis – rock hard, huge and with immense staying power. This, of course, has very little to do with the performance of a real penis, which – like the person to whom it belongs – has its good days and mediocre days. Quite often, though, men develop a distorted idea of their penis size. Comparisons with other men are inevitable but not always reliable. When men see each others' bodies, in communal showers or changing rooms, they see the full dimensions of the penises on display. However, when a man looks down at his own penis, he is going to see it from a different and rather fore-shortened angle. The best way to gauge your true penis size is to look at it sideways in the mirror.

Another anxiety for a man is whether a small penis will make a difference to the pleasure he can give a woman. It should be remembered that width is more important than length in stimulating the lining of the vagina, and thereby giving sexual satisfaction to a woman. The vagina is around 10cm/4in in length, so it is the right size for most penises. In exceptional cases, where an erect penis is very small, it may produce less stimulation. The woman, however, can still be stimulated orally, manually, and in lots of other exciting ways. The vast majority of women would say they fall in love with the man and not his penis. The skill with which a man uses his penis in lovemaking, his degree of sensuality and his sensitivity to her body's responses is what matters most.

▶ *Penises do vary considerably in length, thickness and shape when they are flaccid but these differences become less pronounced once they are erect. A smaller penis will grow proportionally more than a large penis on arousal.*

human complement – including the X or Y chromosomes that will dictate the sex of the embryo after an egg has been fertilized. The mid-section acts as the motor, causing the tail to lash from side to side, thereby propelling the sperm on its journey through the cervix and uterus and into a Fallopian tube in search of an egg. When conditions are right, sperm can survive for several days inside a woman's repro-ductive tract.

Circumcision

A circumcised penis is one in which the foreskin has been surgically removed. This is usually performed for religious reasons, particularly within the Jewish and Muslim communities, or for medical or health reasons. In the case of Jewish children, circumcision is usually carried out when a boy is eight days old. It is usually performed later with

The Circumcised Penis

▼ *Circumcision may be carried out on medical grounds, but more often it is for reasons of hygiene or religion.*

A Spermatozoon

▶ *Despite its microscopic size, a sperm is able to travel a relatively huge distance through the female reproductive tract, propelled by the whip-like action of its tail.*

mid-section

head

tail

nucleus

Muslim children, between the ages of three and 15 years. In western coun-tries, circumcision is more likely to be performed for its perceived health benefits – some people believe the removal of the foreskin reduces the risk of infection as the penis can be more easily kept clean. Circumcision is sometimes carried out for medical disorders such as phimosis, a condition in which the foreskin is too tight to retract prop-erly, or balanitis, in which the tip of the penis becomes inflamed as a result of a buildup of secretions under the foreskin.

The Development of Male Sexuality

Puberty is the time when the male sexual characteristics become fully developed, leading to many changes in a young man's body. The first signs of puberty usually appear later in males than in females, between the ages of 12 and 14 years, although in

some individuals it may be slightly earlier or later than this.

As with girls, the initial changes are triggered by chemical and nerve signals in the hypothalamus, a region of the brain. These signals trigger the release of gonadotrophins which, in turn, instruct the testicles to start releasing increasing levels of male hormones, or androgens, such as testosterone, into the blood stream. These hormonal changes bring about a sudden spurt in bone and muscle development.

The initial signs of puberty in a boy are an increase in the size of the scrotum and testes, followed by the growth of pubic and facial hair. Sperm begins to develop within the testes, and other structures, such as the seminal vesicles and the prostate gland, begin to mature. Around the age of 13 years the penis begins to enlarge, taking around two years to reach its full adult size. The voice also begins to "break" as the larynx

◀ *The development of the man's secondary sexual characteristics is triggered by signals from the hypothalamus, inside the brain, and by hormones from the pituitary gland, just underneath. These stimulate the production of the male sex hormones, such as testosterone. The physical changes are only slight at first, but they speed up during the adolescent years, before stabilizing by the time the male has reached his early twenties.*

▶ *During the adolescent years the male body develops its characteristic shape. Bones lengthen and strengthen, muscles enlarge, and the shoulders broaden as the youth begins to exhibit the physical strength of the adult male. There is usually a dramatic growth spurt between the ages of ten and 16 years, sometimes as much as 17cm/7in in a single year.*

enlarges and the vocal cords thicken and lengthen, causing the voice to drop in pitch.

Body hair appears under the arms and on the chest, and the skin becomes coarser and may darken a little. The increased levels of testosterone tend to overstimulate the oil-producing glands in the skin, leading to acne. This can usually be treated medically and will improve with age. It is not uncommon for an adolescent male to experience temporary breast enlargement. This normally subsides within a few months, though the episode may embarrass him.

Becoming A Man

Puberty can be a difficult time for a young man: he has to come to terms with physical changes in his body, in addition to defining his role as a male in society. He experiences peer group pressure, while trying to live up to the expectations of parents and teachers, yet at the same time he is trying to determine his own beliefs and goals. During this period he may start testing or challenging authority figures as he struggles to assert his own identity. At this stage of a young adolescent's development he will greatly benefit from the friend-

ship and guidance of older men who can act as role models and be prepared to advise him through this difficult, demanding, and changing period of life.

Male Sexual Experience

In addition to physical changes, a young male will probably start to experience exciting but somewhat frightening new sexual feelings. Erections occur frequently, and often at the most inopportune times. In his early teenage years, the adolescent may start to ejaculate during his sleep. These nocturnal emissions are commonly known as "wet dreams".

He will probably also engage in frequent masturbation, fuelled by his awakening desires and his growing fantasies about sex. It is not uncommon for adolescents to engage in sexual play with other boys of the same age. They may compare penises and frequency of ejaculations, and even masturbate together. For most boys this is only a passing phase, and can provide an important means of gaining knowledge about their own bodies and of comparing their development with others.

As a young man gains confidence in himself, he will start to develop an interest in the opposite sex and begin to form relationships. It is just as important for young men to be well informed on subjects such as contraception, sexually transmitted diseases, and the relationship between sexuality and emotional happiness as it is for their female counterparts.

Adolescence is usually a time of sexual experimentation and normally, while the emotions involved may be intense, these relationships do not always last long. In western cultures particularly, young men often feel under peer-group pressure to lose their virginity as soon as possible. According to recent studies of sexual behaviour in Britain, the majority of men claim to have lost their virginity at around the ages of 16 or 17 years. This, of course, is not true for all men, and many males remain virgins until they are much older.

As a boy becomes a man he has to cope with demands made upon him from many different directions. During early adulthood his prime concerns will centre around his studies or career, and establishing himself in his chosen lifestyle, but his relationships with women will also be of great importance.

Man's Sexual Peak

If a man's sexual peak is measured in terms of frequency of orgasm (either through masturbation or lovemaking) and the amount of resting time he needs between each

A Man's Sexual Experiences

▶ *During adolescence, a young man may want to experiment with a number of relationships, and this can help him to build up a broad range of sexual and emotional experiences. As he grows older, however, he will be more inclined to seek his true mate.*

ejaculation, he is at his most sexually potent in the years of late adolescence and early twenties. Generally, after that age his virility stabilizes, and then declines slightly in later years as he requires longer periods of recovery between each ejaculation. However, most men improve their lovemaking skills as

they get older, acquiring more knowledge about their own physical responses and becoming more sensitive to a woman's sexual needs. So, in fact, age can make a man a better lover, with more staying power during coitus. This undoubtedly enhances his sexual satisfaction, both physically and emotionally.

The Pleasure Zones

There are many pleasure zones in the sexual geography of the human body. When directly stimulated by touching, kissing, nuzzling, nibbling and licking they can awaken and heighten sexual response. Most sexually experienced adults know about the principle erogenous areas, such as a woman's lips, breasts, and clitoris, and a man's lips and penis. But a careful and caring lover also takes time to discover the more secret and mysterious pleasure sites on a partner's body.

It is important to think of your lover's body as a complete and integrated organism, of which every inch is worthy of loving attention and caresses, rather than as a map where specific areas are singled out for erotic arousal. Nothing is more of a turn-off than a text-book lover who has read all the information, and then proceeds to focus on a few selected parts of the body, to twiddle and fiddle with the expectation of scoring a sexy result.

Knowing the erotic physiology of the body is just one aspect in understanding and satisfying your lover's sexual needs. Whatever part of the anatomy you stimulate with your fingers, tongue, lips, breasts or penis, you simultaneously touch and arouse the emotional psyche of your partner.

The body's pleasure areas differ from one person to another, so the best way to discover the most erotically susceptible places on your partner's body is with foreplay, when you can lovingly, teasingly and sensitively explore each other from top to toe.

Do not be afraid to ask how and where your lover most likes to be touched, and what kind of stimulation brings the greatest sexual thrill.

You should also try to learn more about your own body's erotic responses, for this can be a changing and ongoing process of discovery.

Touch games and sensual massage techniques are also excellent ways to become familiar with one another's physical needs and responses, while regular tactile stimulation of the skin's sensory system will heighten its erogenous reactions.

Common Erogenous Zones in Both Sexes

Men and women differ in the way they respond to erotic tactile stimulation. Women tend to need more whole body touch to reach the height of sexual arousal, and are generally more sensitive to skin sensations than are their male partners.

It is highly possible for a woman to reach orgasm purely through the oral or tactile stimulation of her breasts, nipples or mons. Men, on the other hand, are greatly aroused by visual stimulation, and are much less likely to reach orgasm without direct physical contact with the penis, their most erogenous zone.

Loving Signals
▲ *Words of love, praise and affirmation, the look of appreciation in your eyes, your patience and understanding of your lover's unique sexuality, are as important to the art of lovemaking as your knowledge of a partner's erogenous zones.*

Sexual Fine Tuning
▶ *Tuning in to your partner's body is like learning to play a fine musical instrument. You need to become sensitive to all its subtle nuances.*

Fun of Discovery
▶ *The entire body is a potential pleasure zone for you to have fun exploring.*

Some of these differences are the result of cultural conditioning; women are much more encouraged to enjoy their total sensuality, while men are taught to focus purely on their genital sexuality.

Most men who allow themselves to experience and enjoy a softer and more sensual approach to lovemaking will discover the sheer joy and eroticism which exists in whole body touch. Both sexes will respond well

Sexual Nuzzling
▲ *Nibbling and nuzzling the soft sensual areas of the face is very sexy. Include the ears, nose and lips.*

Passionate Kisses
▼ *Trace the fullness of the lips with your tongue, and kiss the mouth gently, allowing the passion to increase before penetrating with your tongue.*

Teasing Tongue

▼ *Stroke the belly gently as you cover it with slow and teasing kisses, then run your tongue around his nipple.*

Playful Nibbling

▼ *Toe nibbling is a playful pursuit and, especially when concentrated on the big toe, can be a major turn-on.*

to loving attention on the following parts of the body:

Head and face: Tenderly caress and kiss the forehead, brows, eyelids, tip of the nose and the chin. Comb your fingers through the hair and plant tiny kisses along your partner's hair-line.

Neck and shoulders: Nibble and kiss along the sides and down the back of the neck and shoulders to send electric shivers through the body.

Belly and navel: The belly is a vulnerable but sexually exciting area because of its close proximity to the genitals. Rub your face softly against the belly and then blow gently over it. Cover it slowly and teasingly with kisses, and slide your tongue around the navel, before travelling slowly down to the pubic area.

Perineum: This area extends from the external genitalia towards and including the anus. It is richly served with highly erotic nerve endings and sensitive hair follicles. Stroking over the perineal skin and around the anal rim can greatly enhance sexual excitement.

Legs and thighs: Stroke the legs to awaken the sensuality of the lower half of the body. Focus on the thighs, particularly the inner leg, trailing your fingertips towards the groin. The backs of the knees are surprisingly sensitive to erotic touch. Brush your lips against the skin, and let your tongue travel over it in circular movements.

Feet and toes: Squeeze and knead the feet to activate their many nerve endings and so bring them alive. Toe sucking, and rolling your tongue over the webs of soft skin between the toes can be a powerful sexual turn-on. (Always make sure that the feet are clean and the skin is healthy first.)

The Miracle of the Skin

The skin is our largest sensory and erotogenic organ. It houses our sense of touch, and its sensitivity and importance to our survival is second only to the brain and the central nervous system. In fact, during our initial development in the womb, the skin, the sense organs, and the central nervous system are produced from the same ectoderm tissue, the outermost of the three layers that make up the early embryo form.

In this way the skin can be seen as the external, feeling surface of the internal mental processes of the brain. It has a vast network of nerve endings which responds to all manner of stimuli, from pain to pleasure. These impulses are transmitted through the nervous system to the brain.

Some areas of the skin, such as the breasts, nipples, lips, and genitals, as well as other more surprising parts of the body, are richly supplied with a high density of exquisitely sensitive and erotogenic nerve endings, sending signals of sexual pleasure to the brain and back to the entire body.

As sexual arousal grows during foreplay and intercourse, the breathing becomes deeper and the tissues get infused with oxygen. This increases the excitability of the nerves at the surface of the skin, especially around the genitalia, so that the body becomes even more sensitive to touch. It is through this process of tactile stimulation, particularly to the most erogenous areas of the body, that men and women are brought to the very peak of sexual pleasure and so reach orgasm.

A Woman's Erogenous Zones

The arms and hands: Kiss her hands and wrists tenderly and then suck gently on the fingertips. Pay attention to the soft skin on the underside of the arm, letting your mouth slowly move up towards the armpit.

Breasts and nipples: Treat them gently and with great respect. The breasts are glands, not muscles. This intimate area is packed with highly erotogenic nerve endings, which are directly connected to the emotional centres of her brain. Slowly and deliciously stimulate them with your fingers and tongue.

Thighs: Lick, kiss or stroke the thighs, especially along the soft skin of the inner thigh muscles and around the groin.

Mons pubis: The pubic area is a highly erotogenic area on a woman's body, with a rich supply of nerve endings at the base of the hair follicles. Gently rub or tug on the pubic hairs.

Clitoris: Every man should know more about a woman's clitoris as it is undoubtedly the most sexually important organ in her body, packed with highly erotogenic and sensitive nerve endings to the same extent as a man's penis. Focus on the clitoris only when her whole body has become sexually alive and receptive, and then caress it with your tongue and fingers to bring her to the peak of sexual arousal. Watch out for her signals indicating whether she wants you to change from gentle caresses to more vigorous stimulation.

A Man's Erogenous Zones

Chest and nipples: Stroke his chest and pectorals with your hands, and run your tongue around his nipples before sucking them gently. As with a woman, this area is sensitive to erotic arousal.

Penis and scrotum: Too much premature attention here could bring him to ejaculation too soon, as this is the most sexually charged area of a man's body. Run your hands and tongue playfully over his penis and scrotum, and cover them with tender and tantalizing kisses, before moving down his body.

Buttocks: Focus attention on his buttocks, a very sexually charged zone for men, packed with erogenous nerve endings. Knead and squeeze the fleshy area firmly with your hands.

Back of the body: Men are aroused by sensual touches on the back of the body. Stroke his shoulders and run your fingers down his spine, and then caress his calves and the back of his thighs.

Nipple Caresses
▲ Run the tip of your tongue around the areola, the dark pigmented area surrounding the nipples. Suck gently on the nipple and then dart your tongue back and forth over its tip.

Back Strokes
▲ Use long, languorous, caressing touches on the shoulders and along the spine, before making gentle stroking movements over the backs of the legs.

Chapter 3

Sex Awareness

Sexual vitality depends on both emotional and physical relaxation, and an inner sense of harmony between body, mind and spirit. Sexuality does not function as something separate from who we are, but is an expression of all the aspects of our inner and outer being. By affirming a healthy image of ourselves, through visualization, positive thinking and self-affirmation, we can transform negative thoughts which function from the subconscious mind into positive ones to affect the way we relate to ourselves and others in a beneficial way. Breathing techniques, pelvic exercises, either alone or with a partner, will help emotional and sexual tensions to release as muscles become more relaxed. Learning to love and self-pleasure our bodies is now regarded as a positive step towards gaining emotional and sexual health. Make these occasions sensual and luxurious so that you are able to explore and discover your full sexual responses.

Sexual Health Awareness

Sexual health awareness is about developing a deeper understanding of the sexual self and discovering how the mind and body interact to achieve true fulfilment. It involves a commitment to a regular health regime, to include sexual hygiene, medical check-ups and a programme of physical and mental exercises, as well as an awareness of the sexual body and of the way it changes and develops at different stages throughout life. By following a sexual health awareness programme you can learn how to become attuned to your basic physical, emotional and psychological needs, thus helping you to achieve more satisfying and fulfilling relationships and a feeling of personal well-being.

The first step towards sexual health awareness is the confidence that comes with the knowledge that your body is clean and wholesome and free from illness and disease. This will help you to feel more relaxed in mind and body and boost your self-esteem because you will be able to feel assured that you are physically appealing to the opposite sex.

Your sexual health routine should include an understanding of the way your sexual body looks and feels on a day-to-day level so that medical disorders, if they arise, are identified at an early stage, when they can be more easily treated. This approach is particularly important for a woman because the hormonal fluctuations that routinely occur throughout the menstrual cycle cause physical changes which may mask possible medical disorders unless she is totally in tune with the many different facets of her body.

Sexual Hygiene for Women

The sense of smell is powerfully evocative and so it is to be expected that many women feel self-conscious about their natural aroma. In fact, this is an exaggerated worry as a woman's basic scent is a potent turn-on for men and does not need to be masked by pungent fragrances and perfumes. Plain water and a mild unscented soap are perfectly adequate for daily washing.

Many women are over-zealous about their sexual hygiene, often scrubbing too vigorously and using highly scented, antiseptic soaps, bath salts and bubble baths. These preparations can cause skin irritation and may even lead to an allergic reaction in serious cases. It is only necessary for women to wash the external part of the genitalia, as the vagina itself is self-cleansing. In particular, douches or vaginal deodorants are to be avoided, except on medical advice, as these can irritate the vagina's sensitive lining, and upset its delicate bacterial and chemical balance. This can lead to conditions such as thrush (candidiasis).

The most important sexual hygiene rule is to always wash the bottom from front to back, to avoid spreading infection. If you use flannels, keep one solely for the genital/anal area, be sure to wash it out after use and leave it open on a radiator to dry thoroughly. A damp flannel provides a perfect breeding ground for germs.

Flush Out Infection

▶ *Cystitis, or inflammation of the bladder, is a common and distressing problem for many women and is often caused by infection spreading up through the urethra. At the first sign of an attack, you should drink a large glass of water and repeat this every three to four hours to flush out the bacteria.*

It is important to learn the look and pattern of your normal vaginal secretions so that you can recognize if an abnormal pattern develops. These secretions usually increase during sexual arousal and at the mid point in the menstrual cycle, around the time of ovulation. If you develop a discharge that seems out of the ordinary, particularly if it is accompanied by soreness or itching of the genital area, it may indicate an infection, and you should see a doctor as soon as possible.

Signs of infection include a copious watery secretion that is greenish or greyish in colour, possibly with a fishy smell, or a discharge that has the creamy consistency of cottage cheese. Other signs include sores, inflammation, rash, pain in the lower abdomen, pain or discomfort when urinating, and blood in the urine. You should avoid having sex until the condition has been identified and successfully treated.

Some sexually transmitted diseases cause symptoms in men but not in women, although they may still lead to infertility or other serious conditions. If a sexual partner complains of symptoms such as difficulty urinating or abnormal discharge from the penis, encourage him to see his doctor and also seek medical advice yourself.

Because the urethra, the tube that carries urine out of the body, is so much shorter in women they are at much greater risk of infections spreading to the bladder, causing the painful condition cystitis. Sufferers develop a pain in the lower abdomen and find urination painful. In severe cases the urine may be cloudy and the woman may feel feverish. Cystitis can also be caused by soaps, gels, and deodorants and even by bruising as a result of over-enthusiastic lovemaking.

Always see your doctor if the symptoms are severe or persist for longer than a few days as the condition may lead to kidney infection, if left untreated. In the meantime, drink plenty of fluid, and ask your doctor to recommend a suitable painkiller. A hot-water bottle held against the abdomen may help to ease the pain. If you do not suffer from high blood pressure, drinking a solution of baking powder (sodium bicarbonate) can reduce the acidity in the urine and ease the stinging as well as helping to flush out any bacteria.

Breast Care

Caring for your breasts should be an important part of your sexual health regime. Managing your stress levels, and keeping to a diet that is low in saturated fats and refined sugar is thought to promote healthy breasts. Exercise can help strengthen the underlying muscle and so help prevent sagging, although the best way to keep breasts firm is to wear a well-fitting support bra, particularly when playing sport, or during pregnancy and when breastfeeding.

Change your bra size as often as seems necessary and be sure to try a bra on before you buy it. A surprising number of women wear a bra that does not fit properly. After washing your breasts, pat them dry with an upward motion to prevent sagging and use a moisturizer to help keep the skin smooth and supple – again using upward movements.

The breasts usually become slightly enlarged in the second half of the menstrual cycle, mainly as a result of hormonal changes, giving a sensation of heaviness and fullness. They may also feel lumpy. One third of women suffer breast tenderness as a result of these hormonal changes, which can make many activities, including sport, lovemaking and even walking up stairs, very uncomfortable. A common cause of this is

Caring for your Breasts
◀ *Breasts are a major sexual characteristic and are central to a woman's femininity. Learn to examine your breasts regularly for lumps or any signs of change, and use a rich cream moisturizer to help keep the skin supple. To avoid sagging, use an upward motion, as you would on your face.*

benign breast disease (see below), but the pain may also be due to a bruised or strained chest muscle.

Self-help measures include cutting down on stimulant drinks, such as tea or coffee, and taking evening primrose capsules and vitamin B6 (pyridoxine) in the second half of the menstrual cycle. Wearing a support bra day and night might also help. If the pain persists, or affects one side only, you should see your doctor.

Breast Awareness

Breast cancer is the most common form of cancer in women and is most likely to be successfully treated if it is diagnosed at an early stage. Many breast cancers are first detected by the woman herself, so it is important to get to know the normal shape and feel of your breasts throughout the menstrual cycle so that you can spot problem lumps, if they appear.

It is important to remember, however, that benign, or harmless, breast lumps are far more common than malignant, or cancerous, ones. The most common type of lump is a cyst in a blocked gland or duct. Such lumps are most likely to occur in the second half of the menstrual cycle and they usually subside completely after a while.

Monthly lumpiness which does not go away, especially if it is tender,

Breast Self-Examination

Get into the habit of carrying out a monthly breast examination. If you menstruate, a good time to do this is a week after the first day of your period. Undress to the waist and, with your arms at your sides, inspect your breasts in the mirror, from the side as well as the front. Look for any changes of appearance, such as changes in the outline, puckering or dimpling of the skin (like orange peel). Squeeze the nipple to check for bleeding or discharge.

Next, raise your hands over your head and look to see if any puckering or dimpling appears. Put your hands on your hips and push, again looking for puckering or dimpling.

Now, examine your breasts while lying down on the bed. Place a folded towel under one shoulder and raise your arm on that side above your head to stretch the breast. With the flat of the hand only, gently feel the breast using a circular movement and working from the outer edge to the nipple. Also feel for lumps under the armpit. Repeat with the other breast.

is called benign breast disease. This condition, although harmless, may be very painful. Another form of benign breast lump is a fibroadenoma, or fibrous tumour, which is sometimes known as a "breast mouse" because it can be moved around in the breast tissue. A malignant lump is usually not tender and is not mobile.

Because the breasts alter in size and lumpiness throughout the menstrual cycle, it is important to examine your breasts regularly so that you become familiar with these changes. All breasts have normally lumpy areas – so try to discover what is normal for you. During a shower or bath is a good time, particularly when the breasts are soapy.

In addition, at least once a month, you should examine your breasts more systematically. Aim to do this at the same time in your menstrual cycle. A week after the first day of your period is a good time, when the breasts are least lumpy and so easier to check. Look at your breasts in a mirror, in profile as well as from the front, looking for lumps, puckering or dimpling, or any changes in the size or shape.

Other signs include a nipple that has suddenly become inverted, or bleeding from the nipple, or a discharge that is unconnected with breastfeeding. Examine your breasts with your arms raised and then by your sides. If you notice any abnormalities, contact your doctor as soon as possible. If a lump does turn out to be malignant there is a far better chance of a cure if it is detected early.

Medical Screening for Women

Many conditions affecting women can be diagnosed early through regular medical screening checks. One of the most important of these is a cervical smear test which can detect cells that will become cancerous before other signs would become apparent. Treatment at this pre-cancerous stage is fairly simple and has a high success rate. During a smear test, a thin layer of cells is scraped from the cervix and smeared onto a glass slide so they can be examined under a microscope. If abnormal cells are found there will be follow-up tests and, if necessary, treatment.

Doctors recommend that women have a cervical smear test at least every three years. But those in high-risk groups should have annual tests. Women most at risk include those suffering from genital warts (or whose partners have the condition), smokers, and those with multiple sexual partners or who began an active sex life at an early age.

Smear tests are often carried out during routine gynaecological check-ups. During the examination, the doctor will look at the external genital area and into the vagina to check for signs of infection or other abnormalities. The doctor will also feel the lower abdomen to detect possible swelling or tenderness which might indicate a disorder.

Women should also have a breast examination by their doctor at least every three years, if under 40, or annually, if older. Women over the age of 50 are usually screened for breast cancer every three years using a form of X-ray called mammography. However, this method of screening is less effective in younger women because their breast tissue is more dense and any growths do not show up as clearly on the X-ray.

Sexual Hygiene for Men

While the natural musky male smell is attractive to many women, the basic masculine aroma should not be confused with the odour of an unwashed body, which is a positive turn-off. Fresh sweat has no smell, but after six hours bacteria on the skin acts on sweat causing the release

Bath-Time Checks
◀ *Bathing is a good time for both sensual exploration and making regular health checks.*

of unpleasant odours. A regular shower or bath is necessary, and it is particularly important to wash the anal and genital area daily, or more often if necessary.

Uncircumcised men should take particular care to wash the glans (head of the penis) regularly, pulling back the foreskin to ensure it is really clean. This is necessary to prevent the buildup of an oily secretion called smegma which develops under the foreskin. Smegma is a white substance produced by the sebaceous – or oil-producing – glands under the foreskin that helps it to retract smoothly. Without regular washing, smegma can build up and become a source of infection, which can lead to inflammation of the glans, a condition known as balanitis. It has also been linked with cancer of the penis and may cause cervical cancer in partners.

Men should also be alert to any signs which could indicate a sexually transmitted disease, or other serious condition. Signs of infection include pain or discomfort when urinating, abnormal discharge from the penis, or inflammation, sores or a rash around the genitals. It is important to seek medical advice immediately if you notice any of these signs because delay can lead to a worsening of the condition and risks infertility. Abstain from sex until the condition has been identified and successfully treated.

Testicular Awareness

Just as women should learn to recognize the normal shape and feel of their breasts so that abnormalities can be detected straight away, men should get into the habit of examining their testicles regularly so that they can spot a cancerous growth or other problem as early as possible and increase the likelihood of effective treatment.

Testicular cancer is one of the most common cancers in men in the 20–34 age range. It does not usually cause any pain in the early stages and so self-examination is vital if it is to be detected. However, most lumps turn out to be benign conditions, such as a harmless cyst.

You should not notice any pain during the examination, provided you are not squeezing too hard, but if there is discomfort, especially if you notice any swelling, you should seek medical advice. There are several conditions that could cause pain and

Testicular Self-Examination

Make a point of examining your testicles once a month while you are having a bath or shower. Ensure the scrotum is well-covered with soapy lather and then roll each testicle gently between the fingers of both hands. Learn to recognize its normal shape and consistency. Carefully probe for any pea-sized lumps, or nodules, or any swelling or other changes. After your bath or shower, stand in front of a full-length mirror, hold your penis up out of the way and carry out a visual inspection of your scrotum looking for any change in size and shape. Be aware of any pain or sensations of heaviness in the groin or lower abdomen. Report any problems to your doctor.

swelling in the testicles, such as infection or injury, which are unconnected with cancer but which may still require treatment.

A simple testicular self-examination (see above) takes only a few minutes and is best carried out during a warm bath or shower while the scrotum is well-covered with soapy lather. The scrotal skin is most relaxed at this time and the lather will make it easier to slide your fingers over the testicles to search for changes in consistency. After your bath or shower, look at your genitals in a mirror to detect any change in size and shape.

Psychological Exercise

A major step towards finding a partner with whom you can truly relate as an intellectual, sexual, and emotional being is to have confidence in your own mental outlook, physical attractiveness, and emotional status. Before you can develop your self-esteem you must first identify and eliminate the negative patterns of behaviour formed by past experiences and replace them with positive and self-enhancing thoughts and attitudes.

Negative patterns of thought and behaviour can often become etched into the unconscious mind as a result of unhappy childhood experiences, broken relationships and unfulfilled hopes and desires. These harmful facets of the human psyche represent a heavy burden, holding us back in our attempts to form loving liaisons based on mutual respect and esteem. Yet we are often totally unaware of the unwelcome mental baggage we are carrying around with us.

The effect that the mind has on our psychological make-up can be likened to an iceberg. It is only our conscious mental processes that we are fully aware of yet these actually play a very small part in the development of our psychological profile. It is the unconscious, an unseen force lurking below the waterline of our awareness, that has the most profound influence on our behaviour patterns, our self-image and

Contemplative Contentment
▶ *Take time to meditate each day to help you unravel the tensions caused by the daily stresses and strains and to restore your spirit to a state of equilibrium. Find a quiet place where you will not be disturbed, and light candles to enhance the meditative atmosphere. Then sit with your back straight, and breathe naturally, focusing your awareness on your breathing as you inhale and exhale.*

our ability to form lasting and meaningful relationships.

Negative patterns of thought that have formed in the unconscious can damage our self-esteem and hinder our attempts to form lasting relationships. By following a daily pattern of psychological exercises we can get in touch with our unconscious selves and repair the damage caused to our sense of self-worth.

Breathing and Meditation

To form a loving and giving relationship with another person you must first learn to be at peace with yourself. Pressures at work, the demands of friends and relatives, as well as the constant reminders of international

tensions, make this increasingly difficult. However, it is vital for your mental equilibrium that you try to set aside some time each day for quiet contemplation in order to relax your mind and body completely.

You have to cut yourself off totally from the turmoil of the outside world until you are able to restore your physical and emotional nature to a state of peace and harmony. You will then be able to return to the pressures of the daily routine feeling revitalized and replenished in body, mind and spirit.

The first step on this road is to learn the correct breathing techniques. Breathing powers the brain cells so that you become more open and alert, it provides the vital nutrients required by the tissues and removes harmful wastes. Correct breathing will recharge your batteries when you are feeling tired and will soothe you when you are feeling anxious or under stress. Don't force your breathing. Inhale and exhale through your nose, letting the air flow smoothly down into your abdomen and feeling it spread throughout your body, replenishing its cells. Close your eyes and focus on your breathing, feeling the rise and fall of your abdomen as you breathe.

Breathing can then combine with meditation to help you relax totally and get in touch with your inner being. Seek out a quiet place to sit and meditate for 20 minutes and make it a daily routine of relaxation. To enhance the contemplative atmosphere, close the curtains, turn down the lights and let candlelight cast a gentle glow.

Make sure you have a comfortable, straight-backed chair to sit on so you can maintain a good upright posture, or sit cross-legged on a cushion on the floor, keeping your back straight. Take a few minutes to relax and then start to breathe regularly, as above. Clear your mind of all thoughts and just concentrate on your breathing, focusing on the slow and regular movements of your abdomen. Now direct your breathing to all areas of the body, relaxing each part in turn with every exhalation. Work slowly from your toes to the top of your head, paying special attention to the legs, pelvis, back, shoulders, arms, neck and head.

By developing these meditation skills you will find a way to get in contact with the innermost reaches of your mental processes and help your psyche to be more receptive in preparation for the next stage of your programme of mental self-improvement – to develop a loving attitude towards yourself.

Positive Thinking

Negative feelings about your physical or psychological self, and indeed whether you are even worthy of forming a good relationship, can act as a self-fulfilling prophecy, either

Accentuate the Positive
▶ *The first step towards finding a loving and fulfilling relationship is to have a positive attitude towards yourself. How can you expect someone else to love you if you don't love yourself?*

blocking attempts to enter into new liaisons, or ensuring that any relationship that develops is full of disharmony and discord and so bound to fail. By following a psychological exercise programme each day you can eliminate negative thoughts and accentuate positive ones. You will not only feel good about yourself but also encourage others to feel the same way about you too, fostering a sense of love and equilibrium in any partnership that develops.

A low self-image can often become deeply ingrained as a result of the negative messages we have received from friends, relatives and loved ones, particularly in our early formative years when we were at our most vulnerable and impressionable. Therefore, if you are to develop a positive image of yourself you must first find a way to counteract these negative feelings.

The Love of Laughter
▲ *Never underestimate the importance of smiling and laughter to lighten up your life. If you make the effort always to look for the joyful aspects of every situation, rather than being suspicious of happy feelings, you will encourage others to share your sparkling mood.*

The first step is to try to identify those aspects of your thoughts and feelings about yourself that embody your negative mental patterns and to write them down as a list on one side of a piece of paper.

These may be, for example: "I am not attractive", "I am not sexually desirable", "I am not worthy of a relationship", "Nobody could love me", "My relationships don't last". Next, on the opposite side of the paper, write down the positive affirmations that counteract these negative images. Write "I AM attractive", "I AM sexually desirable", "I AM worthy of a relationship", "I CAN be loved", "My relationships WILL last".

Say these things to yourself every day and this continual reinforcement of your positive nature will change the negative patterning of your subconscious mind, creating a direct effect on your conscious actions, and your attitudes to others.

Visualization Techniques

When individuals have endured a very painful experience in a relationship, or have been left deeply scarred as a result of psychological trauma, or a broken family background, it can leave them feeling disillusioned with themselves and lacking confidence in their ability to form loving relationships. In such cases they will often have to reach deep down inside their subconscious to undo the damage that has been caused.

One way to achieve this is to use the technique of positive visualization. Sit in front of a large mirror, and make yourself comfortable. You need to be very relaxed, so use the deep-breathing and meditation techniques you have already learnt to get into a relaxed and receptive frame of mind, ensuring that you keep your eyes closed.

Once you feel physically and mentally at peace, cast your mind back to a time when you felt truly

Eliminate the Negative

◀ *You can turn negative thoughts into positive ones by following a programme of exercises for making positive affirmations. Write down those thoughts and judgements you have on yourself, and then counteract them with positive affirmations. Repeat this regularly to yourself to counteract the negative patterning of your thoughts.*

loving towards another person, recalling the situation in minute detail. Try to remember where you were, who you were with, and what had happened to make you feel this way. Recapture the feelings of love that you experienced at the time and fill your mind and body with them.

Now, open your eyes and look at the image of yourself with the feelings of love, tenderness, warmth, and joy you have just re-evoked. Think about the various aspects of yourself that you most admire; not just the physical characteristics that you are happiest with – your attractive eyes, perhaps, your shapely legs, or your long hair – but also the personality traits that you think are most worthy of appreciation – maybe your intelligence, loyalty, perseverance, or perhaps your affectionate tender nature.

Once you have begun to see yourself in this new and affirming light, concentrate on those aspects of your character that you would like to improve. Perhaps you would like to be more relaxed, or more energetic, more forgiving, or more loving. Repeat this exercise every day. You may not get spectacular results immediately, but slowly these positive affirmations will print themselves over the negative patterning that existed before.

By enhancing this positive self-image, you give out a confident, contented aura that encourages others to think highly of you as well, and so increases your chances of forming a successful and fulfilling relationship.

Once you are in a relationship, it is important to continue with these exercises to reinforce your positive thinking patterns and to counteract any discordant feelings that might arise. You can use these techniques with your partner to reinforce each other's self-image and your loving feelings towards one another.

Take it in turns to make positive loving statements about each other while gazing deeply into your partner's eyes. Combine this with mutual breathing and meditation sessions to help bring you closer on an emotional and spiritual level.

Seeking Friendship

To achieve true contentment, it is important to feel fulfilled on all levels. If you are in a committed relationship it is all too easy to look to your partner to satisfy all your emotional and psychological needs. In fact, though, it is rarely possible for one person to gratify another's wants and desires in this way. For example, it might be a very loving and contented partnership on a domestic level, but there may also be major intellectual differences, perhaps one of you is interested in opera or philosophy and the other prefers to talk about sport and listen to pop music.

If you keep looking to each other to fulfil your needs on every strata it can quickly drain the relationship, leading to disharmony and conflict. For this reason it is vitally important to have a wide circle of friends to act as a natural resource from which you can

Fulfilment of Friends

◀ *It is important to have a wide circle of friends outside of a sexual relationship. Friends can provide communication, empathy, and support that comes from shared interests and a similar outlook, and can often satisfy needs that cannot be fulfilled within the sexual relationship itself.*

gather all the mental and spiritual stimulation you need and also to share parts of yourself that perhaps do not flourish within the partnership.

These friends should include members of the same sex to satisfy other aspects of the relationship that your partner cannot give you. The nourishment that comes with this form of close bonding can be very important. In any relationship, certain issues crop up, whether of a sexual, or emotional nature, that you cannot not talk over with your partner, or indeed any member of the opposite sex. In these situations you can greatly bene- fit from talking to someone of the same sex who will have a natural empathy to your situation. Men and women can more easily relate to their own sex and have a common outlook, and a meeting of minds, which could rarely be achieved with a partner, no matter how close. Women are usually much better at forming these sympa- thetic, same-sex relationships, but men, too, can benefit from having friends that they can relate to on an emotional level and who will provide insights and experiences from which they can learn.

Discovering yourself is an ongoing process and one that can never be fully achieved even if you devoted your entire lifetime to the task. But there are a wide range of self- improvement books that help you achieve greater insights into your mental and emotional condition and enable you to fulfil more of your potential. Books on relaxation, visu- alization, meditation and positive thinking, for example, can help to reveal dormant abilities and find new ways to accentuate your latent active and creative sides, while at the same time eliminating the destructive and negative aspects of your nature.

Expand Your Mind

◀ *Self-discovery is an ongoing process. Take time to study self- improvement books and learn to expand your consciousness so that you can release all the potential that is lying dormant deep inside your psyche.*

Exercises for Sexual Fitness

Physical exercises that concentrate on the key sexual areas of the pelvis, lower back, buttocks, abdomen and thighs can release the tension in body and mind that prevents you achieving your full orgasmic potential. These exercises allow you to achieve the strength, suppleness and mobility you need to explore and express fully the physical aspects of lovemaking, and when combined with correctly focused breathing techniques, they open up energy channels in your body which will enhance your enjoyment of sex, and enable you and your partner to achieve a feeling of greater spiritual harmony and union.

Sex is fundamentally a physical activity, so if it is to be enjoyed to the full it is important to ensure that the muscle groups, tendons and joints that come into play during healthy vigorous lovemaking are supple and well conditioned. The positions and movements involved in the various forms of sexual intercourse put muscles and joints under pressure in a way that is totally different from that encountered during routine daily activities.

Unless you keep your body supple and pliant you are liable to suffer muscle cramps and strains during sexual intercourse as you and your partner try to achieve the different angles and changes of position you are seeking in order to obtain mutual sexual satisfaction.

By conditioning the areas of the body that are most actively involved in lovemaking – most notably the muscles of the buttocks, abdomen, thighs, lower back, and pelvic floor – you will extend your range of motion and enhance your ability to move smoothly and with control, enabling a wider variety of pelvic movements and allowing more comfortable lovemaking.

When you are sexually fit you have the suppleness, mobility, and enthusiasm to throw your mind and body into the passion of the moment and even to explore new positions and hitherto undiscovered heights of ecstasy.

By relieving tension you are also helping to fight the stress that often prevents you getting into the relaxed and giving mood needed to achieve a satisfying sexual encounter. Tension in the pelvis, legs, lower back, and abdomen restricts the flow of sexual energy and vitality and reduces your total enjoyment of lovemaking. Repressed feelings here can upset the wholeness and unity of the body and act as a barrier between the mind, the emotions and the physical responses. Exercises combined with breathing techniques, that you can carry out alone or with your partner, will release the tension in these key areas, and help to release the flow of sexual energy so that you can achieve your full orgasmic potential.

Gentle Warm-Up

As with all physical exercises, ensure you are fully warmed up before you try these routines to reduce the risk of minor strains and sprains. Exercise is best carried out after a warm bath or shower so that relaxing warmth is

Pelvic Swing

▼ Stand with your feet a shoulder-width apart, knees slightly flexed. Place your arms by your side with your palms open forwards. Breathe in and draw your pelvis back.

▼ Breathe out and swing your pelvis forwards, allowing arms, hands and genitals to swing up. Repeat this for up to five minutes as a continuous pelvic motion.

transmitted deep into the muscle fibres. Put on some loose, comfortable clothing, choose a room that is draught-free and fairly warm (but not too warm), and ensure you have a soft floor surface to lie on.

Start off the session with some loosening movements and gentle stretches to free the muscles and tendons. Follow this up with ten minutes of vigorous activity, such as brisk walking or a quick jog. Alternatively, try a simple warm-up routine such as marching on the spot while circling your arms above your head. Remember to fill your lungs with air when you start an exercise to ensure your body gets all the oxygen it needs, and then expel your breath on the exertion to rid the body of the waste products it has accumulated.

Pelvic Circles

▼ *Stand with your feet a shoulder-width apart and knees slightly flexed. Place your hands on hips. Mentally focus inside to the inner shape of your pelvic bowl.*

▼ *Rotate your pelvis slowly in wide circles – ten times to the right and then ten times to the left. Breathe in to the movement and consciously allow any tension to relax.*

The following simple routines can help release tension in the abdomen, lower back and pelvis.

Breathing

Correct breathing is a vital part of these exercises. Your breathing is directly affected by your emotional state as a result of external worries

Deep-Breathing Exercise

◄ *Deep breathing brings oxygen to the cells to nourish the body, and eases emotional tension by relaxing the muscles, making you feel more alive and vital. Your partner can kneel behind and encourage the tension to melt by placing his hands softly over the key areas of the chest, diaphragm and abdomen. Breathe into each area in turn, focusing awareness into every inhalation and exhalation.*

and pressures. When you are tense and under stress your breathing becomes rapid and shallow and your body cannot get all the air it needs for normal healthy functioning.

By focusing on your breathing you can draw the air deep down into your abdomen to fill the lungs to capacity. This saturates the blood with life-giving oxygen, which is then pumped round the body to restore the tissues and replenish the energy reserves depleted during physical activity. When you breathe out, aim to empty your lungs completely to rid your body of the waste products that have built up. This slowly releases the emotional tension, leaving you feeling relaxed, more alive and vital.

Pent-up feelings of anger, anxiety, or fear can also lead to tension in the key energy centres of the body – the chest and abdomen. Inhalation and exhalation can be combined with the healing power of touch to help you direct your breathing into each part

Solo Pelvic Release Exercise

▼ *Lie down comfortably on your back and place your hands over your abdomen. Close your eyes and breathe slowly and deeply into your belly, then slowly breathe out, emptying your lungs as you do so. Notice your abdomen softening and expanding with each inhalation, feel it fall back with each exhalation. Imagine the whole area is relaxing with each outward breath.*

in turn, to unblock the energy channels and release the sexual tension.

Place your hands softly over the chest and abdomen and imagine that the warmth and contact of your hands is melting these areas.

Encourage the tension to drain away as you focus your awareness into every inhalation and exhalation. You can do these exercises by yourself, sitting or lying down, or encourage your partner to sit behind you resting his hands gently on your chest and abdomen.

Strengthening the Pelvic Floor

You can greatly enhance your sex life by learning exercises to strengthen the pelvic floor. This is the collection of muscles and ligaments at the base of the abdomen that supports the bladder, vagina, uterus, and rectum. Childbirth and ageing can weaken this part of the body, reducing control over the vaginal and pelvic muscles and blunting the nerve responses. A weakened pelvic floor can also lead to serious medical problems such as a prolapsed uterus and urinary incontinence and is often the underlying cause for women who are having difficulty achieving an

Genital Release Exercise with Partner

This exercise releases sexual tension in the pelvic and genital area and increases vitality. Lie down comfortably on your back, with your feet on the ground and knees raised. Your partner gently supports your head. Place your hands over your chest and abdomen to encourage breathing and aid relaxation. Repeat this exercise for up to five minutes, then rest for five minutes – feel the vibrations in your legs and body and acknowledge any rising feelings.

▲ *Breathe into your chest and abdomen. Imagine your breath to be reaching your genitals. Breathe in and out.*

▲ *Place your arms by your side. Breathe in – draw your thighs together. Imagine your in-breath to be pulling your legs in.*

▲ *Breathe out – let your legs flop open – to open up the genitals and relax the thigh muscles and groin. Then breathe in again.*

Squats

▶ *Squat on your haunches, placing your feet wide enough to support your body. Let your buttocks drop down, and relax your anus. Feel your entire pelvic floor relaxing. Breathe in four to five short breaths (don't exhale). With each inhalation, draw up and tighten the pelvic floor muscles, as if pulling your vagina up step by step. Then give five short out-breaths (don't inhale) releasing your pelvic floor muscles step by step. Do this ten times to tone the pelvic floor muscles.*

orgasm. Regular pelvic floor exercises will ensure that these muscles and ligaments remain taut and well toned, so that you have adequate structural support for the uterus and vagina, and will be able to continue to enjoy sex.

Many women also find that by toning up the muscles of the pelvic floor they are able to climax more freely and to experience stronger or more intense orgasms. Improving the strength and flexibility of these muscles will extend your range of movement and make those positions that involve squatting over your partner, or wrapping your legs round him, easier and more comfortable to adopt. Your vagina will also be able to grip your partner's penis more firmly during lovemaking, which will enhance the enjoyment for both of you.

The following exercises will tone and strengthen the pelvic floor. They are particularly important after childbirth, but all women will derive some benefit from them. You will particularly notice the effect during lovemaking when you find that your vagina is better able to clasp your partner's penis – but be careful not to

squeeze too tight! You can discover your pelvic floor by imagining you need to urinate but are trying to hold it back. The part of the body that tightens as you do this is your pelvic floor. In addition to the exercises in this section, there is a simple pelvic floor exercise that you can practise at any time, as no one can see you do it. Slowly contract the pelvic floor muscles, ten times, pulling the muscles up inside in slow stages each time. Breathe normally as you do this exercise. Practise two to three times daily for at least a month. Another exercise you could try on your own is to place two fingers inside the vagina and try to squeeze them by contracting the muscles.

Pelvic Curls

This exercise is good for strengthening the pelvis and thighs – it aids whole-body vitality, improves posture, strengthens support for the vital organs, and relaxes the lower back. Do this exercise five times. Lie with your back on the ground with the whole of the spine touching the floor – including the small of your back. Let the ground support your weight. Keep your knees bent and place the soles of your feet flat on the floor, a shoulder-width apart, supporting your legs. Put your arms by your sides with your hands palms-down on the floor.

▲ *Breathe out and roll your spine upwards, using your buttocks and lower abdominal muscles to curl your tailbone up off the floor. At the same time tighten your buttocks and inside thigh muscles.*

▲ *Now breathe in and roll your spine down to the floor, uncurling your tailbone and relaxing your buttocks and inside thigh muscles.*

Self-Pleasuring

Nowadays, masturbation is regarded by most sex experts as a normal and even beneficial sexual activity. However, until recent times, masturbation was a taboo subject. It was considered immoral, termed a "sin", and young people were warned that it would make them mad, blind, infertile, or ruin their chances of sexual happiness in marriage. Not so long ago, the word "masturbation" was defined as "self-abuse" in a standard dictionary. That view of masturbation has now radically changed.

Attitudes to masturbation began to alter in the late 1940s and early 1950s, when the Kinsey reports on male and female sexuality stated that, according to their studies, 94 per cent of American men and 40 per cent of American women masturbated to orgasm. More recent research suggests that, while the figure for male masturbation remains the same, female masturbation is now considerably higher, though still less than for men.

Masturbation, which is the self-stimulation of one's own genitals for sexual pleasure and orgasm, is clearly, then, a normal part of human sexual activity. None of the dire warnings that were made about it were found to be true. In fact, the Kinsey report concluded that the only harmful side-effects of masturbation were the anxiety and guilt it might evoke in those who practised it.

Masturbation is now seen more as "self-pleasuring" than abuse. It is a valuable way for males and females, young and old, to learn more about their bodies, and to enjoy their sexual and orgasmic responses. It can be a useful way to release sexual tension, but more importantly, it gives men and women the chance to enjoy sexual pleasure and body sensuality, regardless of whether or not they are currently in a relationship.

These days, masturbation is one of the basic tools used in sex therapy, and clients are often encouraged to masturbate in the privacy of their homes as one of the key methods of discovering and encouraging their sexual and orgasmic responses and of overcoming their anxieties, guilt or other problems surrounding sexual issues.

Art of Self-Pleasuring

Masturbation is often carried out in a speedy and rather unsensual fashion, with the aim of achieving a climax in the fastest way possible by focusing the manual stimulation solely on the genital organs. This method has its uses, especially if the aim is to obtain a quick release from sexual tension. However, to turn it into the art of self-pleasuring, you should learn to feel at ease with the situation so that it can become a way of making love to yourself in a wholly sensual way.

Try to create some time for yourself that is dedicated to self-pleasuring. Ensure that you have complete privacy and that you won't be interrupted. Warm your bedroom and light some candles, if it is dark, to create a sensual ambience. Have a bath so that you feel relaxed, and then soothe your skin with a lotion. Play some music that will help you feel sexy, and then lie naked on your bed. Begin to stroke and caress your whole body, including your genital area, but do not at this point focus

Vary Your Strokes

▶ *Experiment with different strokes, pressures and speeds of movement, sliding your hand up and down the whole shaft of the penis, from the base to above the ridge of its head, or focus more on applying pressure to the erotically-sensitive frenulum.*

specifically on it. If you have an imaginative mind, allow your fantasies to unfold, but also remain totally involved in the physical sensations happening in your body as you touch and stimulate yourself.

Self-Pleasuring for Men

Most men, when they masturbate, concentrate the stimulation solely on the penis. Instead, try to let your hands also stroke your chest, belly, thighs, scrotum, perineum and buttocks, sweeping them over your penis as they move from one part of your body to another. If you choose, fantasize that your dream woman is stroking your body, or indulge yourself in whatever imagery works as a powerful aphrodisiac for you.

Uncircumcised men should draw back the foreskin to expose the glans while masturbating. The most erogenously responsive area is usually around the frenulum, on the underside of the shaft, just beneath the head of the penis. Experiment with pressures and strokes, speeds and rhythms, delighting in all the different sensations that you can create.

As your sexual feelings rise, let yourself go, breathing deeply and moving your body, thrusting your pelvis, and making sounds to express your growing excitement. If you feel you are approaching ejaculation, slow down to prolong your self-pleasuring, then build up the tempo towards climax again.

For a truly sensual experience, try to let this pleasuring last for 15 minutes, or even longer, before you climax. As you approach an orgasm, abandon yourself totally to the sensations. Then rest awhile, touching your body and relaxing deeply.

Self-Pleasuring for Women

Women tend to be more naturally sensual in the way they masturbate, and also quite inventive in their style of touching and stimulation. As described above, turn your self-pleasuring into an erotic feast. Prepare your bedroom to make it warm and inviting, so that you can luxuriate in the act of touching and exploring your body. First, though, why not take a bath enhanced by the aroma of aphrodisiac essential oils.

Ylang-ylang, sandalwood, jasmine, rose, basil, patchouli and black pepper are all oils that are sensually and sexually evocative. Choose up to three of any of these oils, mixing a maximum of seven drops in the water, and then relax in the warmth and fragrance of the bath.

When you have dried yourself and used moisturizer on your skin, lie on the bed and allow your erotic fantasies to take over. Touch and stroke your body, including your genital area, thighs, breasts and nipples. As you become mentally and physically aroused, apply different pressures and strokes of your hands and fingers to your pubic and genital

Enjoy Your Body

▲ *Many women touch and caress their whole bodies while they are masturbating. Try stroking and caressing your most erogenous zones, such as your breasts and nipples, to experience a new intensity of sexual arousal.*

area. You can begin by gently arousing the whole area with a circular motion, placing the heel of your hand on your pubic bone and resting your fingers against your vulva.

As you become aroused, part your vaginal lips with your fingers, and stroke all over the inner folds, around the opening of your vagina, and the area surrounding your clitoris. You may want to pull back the hood of the clitoris to apply pressure on it directly, but if this kind of stimulation feels too intense, rub the skin above and beside it instead.

Experiment with different strokes, vibrations, pressures, and rhythms, finding out exactly which sequence of movements is the most erotic for you. Increase the pressure and speed of

Fingertip Caresses

▶ *Stroke around your vaginal lips and clitoral area, sometimes letting your fingers caress the outer edges of the vagina itself, or slipping into it. As you approach orgasm, increase the pressure and speed of your strokes.*

your touches as your arousal builds, and then, as you approach your climax, maintain a more regular tempo, sustaining pressure on your clitoris throughout your orgasm. Let yourself go into the orgasmic contractions, allowing them to pulsate through your whole body. Moan, sigh or cry out, and move your pelvis to enhance the powerful sensations of your orgasmic release.

For even more arousing sensations, men and women can apply a water-soluble lubrication to their genital area while masturbating. However, avoid oil-based products such as petroleum jelly.

Sex Toys

Many forms of sexual aids can play an important role in helping you to discover your sexual self, and to fulfil your full orgasmic potential. They can enable you and your partner to find new and more exciting sexual sensations and to reach greater heights of orgasmic ecstasy. For some women, in particular, sex aids or masturbation may be the only way that they can achieve sexual release, and therefore have a vital part to play in lovemaking.

Sex toys, or sexual aids, have been used to enhance sexual arousal for thousands of years. Love eggs have been known in China since ancient times. These are small oval or circular objects, often of wood or china, which are inserted into the vagina to produce erotic sensations as the woman walks around. They are available today, although modern love eggs are usually hollow, containing smaller balls or weights inside, and are joined by a length of cord.

Aid to Self-Exploration
▲ *A vibrator can be used if you are not currently in a sexual relationship. Run it around your vulva, or place it just above your clitoris. It can help you explore your orgasmic potential. A vibrator is useful for women who have never been able to climax, as it is certain to produce an erotic response, and this can be used as a basis for further sexual exploration.*

A better known example of a sex aid is the dildo, a kind of artificial penis, which may be fashioned out of wood, china or steel and can be used by both men and women. Some forms of dildo are attached to the groin area by straps so that they can be used by women during intercourse with a partner of the same sex, to emulate the male sexual role, or to perform anal sex on a man. Men, too, can strap on a dildo to obtain what is, in effect, a permanently erect penis.

The modern, and more sophisticated, version of the dildo is the vibrator, which is battery powered and contains a small vibrating motor. The vibrations created by the motor can be intensely arousing, particularly for a woman, because they are more efficient at stimulating the sensory nerve endings in the skin that produce sexual excitement and orgasm than normal skin-to-skin contact.

During penetrative intercourse, for instance, sexual stimulation is

Hygiene
Never share sex toys, and always keep them clean by washing them regularly in hot soapy water. A vibrator can be covered with a condom which is thrown away afterwards. If you use a vibrator for anal stimulation, always wash it before inserting it into the vagina, to avoid spreading infection, or keep a vibrator solely for this purpose.

brought about by the friction caused by the penis rubbing along the inside of the vagina and against the labia and clitoris. This triggers the nerve endings at a steady rate and may lead to orgasm. The vibrator, however, can stimulate the nerve endings at a much faster rate, so an orgasm is almost guaranteed.

Sexual Self-Discovery
For a woman to explore her body thoroughly, to find its most sexually sensitive areas, and to reach her orgasmic potential, a vibrator can be an invaluable aid to self-discovery. Vibrators have helped many women to achieve an orgasm for the first time, particularly in those whose enjoyment of sex is hindered by feelings of shame, guilt or embarrassment instilled in childhood.

The intensity of the stimulation from a vibrator can also overwhelm those psychological blocks that may be preventing some women from achieving satisfaction, forcing them to surrender to the pure animalistic pleasure of self-gratification. They can then build on this experience by incorporating the vibrator into their sex sessions with a partner until the remaining mental barriers have been eliminated entirely. Because of guilt feelings, some women may even be reluctant to touch themselves directly to achieve sexual satisfaction, but able to overcome this aversion with a vibrator.

For other women, the inability to achieve sexual fulfilment may be due to their lack of understanding of their

Vibrating Waves of Pleasure
▲ *Introduce a vibrator to sex sessions with your partner. He can use it on you to produce multiple sexual sensations. It will send shock waves of pleasure through your vulva while he kisses and licks your nipples, driving you into a sexual frenzy.*

own sexuality. Here again, a vibrator can be used to discover which parts of the body are erotically sensitive: not only the most obviously erogenous zones, such as the nipples, vagina or clitoris, but other areas, such as the thighs, belly, earlobes, and arms.

You may feel happier if you are alone for your first experience with a vibrator. In that case you should aim to create the right atmosphere in which to explore your body so you can really relax and let yourself go. Choose a time when you will not be disturbed, lock the door, take the phone off the hook, and turn the lighting down low. Revel in your sexual fantasies and let the vibrator do the work. You can play the vibrator over the inside of the thighs and over the mons before slowly running it along the inside of your labia.

Some women may find that the stimulation is too intense if the vibrator is held directly against the clitoris for very long, but if placed just above or alongside, the erotic sensations it produces may be sufficient for them to climax. If you prefer you can

insert the vibrator into your vagina, as a surrogate penis, either moving it in and out to simulate intercourse, or just letting the vibrations have their effect by themselves.

Some women may find that they need additional lubrication if they are going to use the vibrator inside their vagina. Lubricating cream or gel smeared over the labia and clitoris also enhances the sensation when stimulating these areas as well.

Vibrators for Men
A vibrator can heighten a man's sexual response too, although he will probably need some additional manual stimulation to achieve orgasm. For some men, the glans, or tip, of the penis may be too sensitive to take this degree of stimulation for long. However, other men may find it is sufficiently arousing to enable them to reach orgasm, and it has been successfully used to cure impotence in many cases.

The whole shaft of the penis is responsive to the vibrations, particularly the underside and the frenulum. But a vibrator can also be used to discover other highly charged areas on the man's body. The base of the penis is particularly sensitive to the vibrations, and applying the vibrator to the perineum, the area of skin between the anus and the genitals, enables the pulsing effect to reach down to the prostate, a gland that

Erotic Charge
◀ *Use it on your man to show him just how erotically sensitive the male skin can be. Play it over his thighs and buttocks, working teasingly towards his anal area. Rest it on the highly charged zone between his legs, just in front of the anus, for an electrifying experience.*

can produce intense sexual feelings itself when stimulated. Pressure applied to this area can sometimes produce an erection, without using any other stimulation.

Mutual Fun
A vibrator is not only useful for self-pleasure, or for those who are temporarily on their own or without a sexual relationship: it can also be used during intercourse to heighten the sexual response. The man can slide it over his partner's thighs and breasts, or around her vulva. A woman can use the vibrator to stimulate her man's thighs and buttocks.

Vibrators are available in a wide variety of shapes and sizes, from sex shops and through mail order catalogues, so it is worth spending time deciding which type is best for you. Many are skin-coloured to look like an erect penis, with a veining effect down the side. They may be made of soft latex to make them feel more penis-like, and some also oscillate up and down or from side to side.

Some vibrators may be perfectly smooth, or covered with a ribbed or grooved pattern, to increase the stimulation, and they can often be adjusted to produce a powerful throbbing or a delicate pulsation. They can also be very noisy, so check before you take one home, if the sound of the vibrations is likely to be a source of embarrassment.

The Basic Positions

There are a number of lovemaking positions in common practice that most couples feel comfortable with. These allow both the man and woman to express themselves sexually in different ways by taking more active or passive roles in the lovemaking, and thereby eliciting a variety of physical and emotional responses. An equal and balanced sexual partnership is capable of sharing the more dominant and submissive roles quite easily, allowing a natural transfer between the two, either within one episode of lovemaking, or on different occasions.

Exploration, experimentation and a sense of humour are important to keep a sexual relationship interesting and alive. Once you feel comfortable and secure with each other, it is worth trying something new to add variety, fun, and excitement to your lovemaking.

Here, we sum up the basic lovemaking positions, and then on the following pages of this chapter, some of the more popular sexual positions assumed by couples in coitus will be discussed in greater detail. In other sections of this book you will find more adventurous positions that you can add to your lovemaking repertoire, as well as ideas on spontaneous and fun lovemaking.

Man on Top

▲ The most commonly practised position for lovemaking is when the man assumes the more active role and moves on top of his partner. This allows face-to-face intimacy and full, front-of-the-body contact. The nature of this position means the man takes the more dominant role, while the female role is more submissive.

Woman on Top

◄ The woman-on-top position enables the couple to swap the more active and passive roles and allows them to experience and express other aspects of their sexuality. The woman has more freedom to move and is better able to control the depth of the man's thrusts and the stimulation she may need to reach orgasm.

Sitting Position

▶ *In this sitting position, the couple can feel equal in their sexual roles as it allows them to embrace each other closely and feel intimately bonded. While their movements are somewhat limited, it is a perfect lovemaking posture for more meditative intercourse.*

Kneeling Back to Front

▼ *This is a variation of the woman-on-top position in which she kneels astride the man's hips with her back turned to him. While it does not have the intimacy and contact of a face-to-face position, it can allow both partners time to surrender deeply to their own sensations of sexual pleasure. The man can also stroke the woman's back and buttocks, or squeeze the buttocks gently to give her extra erotic stimulation.*

The Man-on-Top Position

Intercourse in which the man assumes the more dominant role, on top of the woman, is one of the most commonly adopted sexual positions. However, as an automatic choice it has been challenged in more recent times because sexually liberated women are just as eager to share the active role in sex.

It is popularly known as "the missionary position", a name first given by Pacific Islanders who witnessed the "strange" marital activities of white missionaries – the wife on her back with her husband on top. The islanders preferred to make love with the woman squatting over her man – a position which allowed her to express her sexuality fully. Certainly the "missionary position" would have been the obvious choice whenever the man assumed the dominant role in the partnership, or the woman regarded her sexual role purely as a duty.

That it still remains a popular choice for sexually emancipated couples is probably because it is a very intimate position, in which partners remain face to face and in eye contact, allowing the exchange of tender and arousing kisses, and words of love. In addition, it offers close physical contact between the most erogenous and vulnerable parts of the body, the pubis, abdomen, chest and breasts.

A woman who, on other occasions, enjoys exploring and expressing the more active part of her erotic nature may also enjoy relaxing sexually into the more submissive role, and letting her man take charge. While this position obviously suits a man who prefers to be the active sexual partner, he should also be prepared to explore other postures if his partner so desires.

The advantage of this position for a man is that he has more command over his pelvic movements. His penis is at a comfortable angle to enter the woman's vagina, and he has better control over the depth of its thrusts, which enables him to regulate his pace and rhythm so that he is able to gain the maximum stimulation needed to reach orgasm.

Preparing for Penetration

▼ *When sensual play progresses to intercourse it is a moment of physical and psychological transition for the man and woman. Both need to be ready in body and mind for this deeper level of intimacy and penetration, so it is important to stay in touch with your own and your partner's responses. Don't rush into penetration if either of you is not quite ready for it. If both are fully aroused by the touches, kisses, words and embraces of foreplay, the woman's vulva will have swelled, and her vagina will be secreting its juices, in readiness to receive the penis; the man's penis will be erect and firm, and able to enter her. Emotionally, both should be open and available to each other, as they enter into coitus. To check that the woman is sufficiently lubricated to accept his penis, the man can stroke his fingers over her vulva and vaginal opening, or simply ask her if she is ready for penetration. She may indicate by words, sounds or touch that she wants him to enter her. He can then guide his penis into her vagina.*

Slow Entry

▼ *In this basic man-on-top position, the man is between the woman's legs as his penis begins to penetrate her vagina. She lies on her back, and opens her legs wide to give him room to enter her. Slow and careful manoeuvring will ensure the penis remains in the vagina and does not slip out, which can happen if either tries to move too rapidly before both bodies have adjusted their fit to each other. Many women love a slow entry, when the tip of the penis enters and lingers teasingly just within the vaginal orifice. This can give her further time to relax, emotionally and physically, so that her vagina is flooded with the total desire to be filled. She can also reach down to caress his scrotum and the shaft of his penis, which is waiting to enter.*

Slow Motion

◀ *The man can begin thrusting with shallow actions, moving his pelvis slowly and gently back and forth, and allowing more time for attunement. On arousal, the first part of her vagina constricts, enabling it to grip the penis securely, adding to the pleasurable sensations of friction. However, if the man is in a state of high arousal, he needs to be careful not to overstimulate the erotically sensitive tip of his penis if he is prone to ejaculating too quickly.*

Making it Comfortable

For the woman, the main disadvantages of the man-on-top position are the restrictions to her own pelvic movements and, unless her partner is particularly aware of his actions, the inadequacy of the clitoral stimulation – an important factor if she wishes to be aroused to orgasm.

Other situations can make this position an unsuitable choice. If a woman is suffering from a back condition, she may find that making love in this position will add to the strain. If her partner is much heavier than her, she may feel confined and burdened by the size difference.

A pregnant woman can feel anxious and uncomfortable about having any weight bearing down on her abdomen. Her breasts may feel particularly sensitive to pressure and, in the later stages of her pregnancy, this position may simply be impossible. In all of these cases, if the man is on top of his partner, he should take care not to put all his weight on her.

The man-on-top position puts the onus on the man to perform, and this may not suit him if he is tired or under stress. While he may desire physical intimacy with his partner, at a time like this it is usually preferable if the woman takes the more active role. Also, if the man is prone to premature ejaculation, he would do well to experiment with the woman-on-top positions which may slow him down and give him greater control over this process.

Intimacy in Intercourse

The man should always remain aware of his partner's sexual responses, and ensure that the shared intimacy which inspired the lovemaking is not suddenly abandoned in the heat of

Aiding Mobility

▲ *For a woman, mobility is more difficult when making love in the man-on-top position. She may find it helpful if a pillow is placed beneath her buttocks to tilt her pelvis. This will give her more freedom of hip movement and take the strain away from her lower back. By placing her feet firmly against the mattress, she can use her leg muscles to add leverage to her pelvic motions, to increase sensation for both of them, and to allow greater clitoral stimulation as it rubs against his pubic bone. To avoid pinning her down with his body, the man should support his own weight with his arms and hands, keeping the trunk of his body slightly lifted above her.*

arousal. Unfortunately, some men see penetration as a green light to go, and start thrusting away intent on an orgasm regardless of what is happening to their partners. In other scenarios, a man may be conscious of the woman's needs and start performing a series of mechanical manoeuvres aimed at giving her an orgasm so that he can go ahead and achieve his own. Neither type of behaviour is particularly desirable nor likely to please the woman, because intercourse is not a race or a gymnastic show, or a question of pushing the right buttons to gain an end result. It is all about two people meeting and merging, breathing and moving together, feeling and responding, and abandoning themselves equally to the sheer physical and emotional pleasure of the moment.

Fortunately, recent research shows that most sexually active men, while still considering female sexuality to be something of a mystery, believe that their partner's satisfaction is as important as their own. For many men, giving sexual joy to their women is the best part of making love. According to the studies, the majority of men do believe that intimacy and affection during lovemaking are very important factors in a woman's sexual happiness.

Penetration with Care

◄ *Full penetration can create feelings of vulnerability as well as physical pleasure. These feelings need to be experienced and there is no need to rush ahead into immediate thrusting. It is important, too, that the man thrusts deeply only when his partner is physically and psychologically ready to receive him, or it may cause her discomfort. Initially, she can place her hands on his hips to help control his pelvic movements until she is ready.*

Sex with Sensitivity

▲ *It is important to stay in touch on an emotional level throughout intercourse. Slow down once in a while, and look deeply into each other's eyes. By allowing the intimacy you feel to be expressed, silently or with words, your lovemaking will become deeply satisfying. Women need to feel emotionally nourished as well as physically aroused during the sexual act. Men benefit too if they try to get in touch with their softer and more vulnerable feelings.*

Focusing Inwards

▶ *Some lovers like to keep their eyes open during lovemaking, while others prefer to keep their eyes closed. If your eyes are open, you can take pleasure in looking at your partner's body and watching his or her arousal and responses. Closing your eyes while making love takes you into a different dimension of sensual feeling because you are able to focus on and enjoy the exquisite bodily sensations arising within you. To savour both experiences, switch from one to the*

other, so that sometimes you have a total awareness of your partner, and at other times you have complete awareness of yourself.

Chapter 4

The Art of Romance

Learning to signal your availability for love and romance is an art. The way you dress not only affects your self-esteem but also projects a certain image to draw to you the kind of person you most wish to attract. Knowing the nuances of body language helps you to be more aware of what your actions are saying. When you meet that special person, you begin a tentative and hopeful journey into the first stages of romance and courtship. How you behave towards each other at this point forms the basis for your future relationship. It is a time when you will need to affirm your feelings for the other, while not overwhelming him or her with your needs. Becoming aware of your hopes and expectations will help you through this difficult period of transition as the new relationship deepens into a more intimate bond.

The Language of Clothes

The clothes you wear can say much about your emotional state and feelings of confidence. Both men and women use clothes to broadcast aspects of their personalities, or to create a certain persona with which to impress other people. That slinky "little black number" can bring out aspects of a woman's character that might otherwise have remained dormant. "Power dressing" inspires respect in others and so gives the individual's own confidence a major boost. In comfy leggings, or jeans and a sweatshirt, on the other hand, a person presents a more relaxed and easy-going image.

Dress to Express

Women often wear more revealing clothes when they are feeling confident about their sexuality. Some researchers claim this is most likely to be around the time of ovulation, when a woman is at her most fertile. However a woman can feel sexy at any time, and the clothes she wears will often reflect this mood, accentuating her most attractive characteristics.

It is a common misunderstanding, though, for a man to assume that a woman dresses purely for the effect her clothes will have on the opposite sex. Very often a woman chooses a certain style, even one that is overtly appealing, because she enjoys feeling attractive in her own right and expects to have the freedom to express it. A woman who chooses to wear a figure-hugging dress or even a revealing mini-skirt may be doing so because she favours the style, wants to feel good about the way she looks, and may be just as concerned about making an impression on her female friends as on men. In other words, if a woman is wearing clothes that reveal her body, it does not necessarily signal that she is wanting or expecting to receive uninvited male attention.

Nowadays, a women has a greater sense of her personal freedom, and her wish to express her sexuality without being perceived as a sex object means that men must decode

Party Time

▲ This short, figure-hugging dress says the woman is in the mood for some fun and is not ashamed to broadcast the message. The dress is shaped to reveal the sensual curve of her neck, while the high heels accentuate the length of her legs. By choosing black she is also showing she feels confident and in control.

her availability signals without simply basing them on the way she is dressed. This can be difficult to grasp for a man who is conditioned to believe that a woman's desire to look attractive is only designed for a male response. These days, if a woman wishes to attract the attention of a man, she is likely to give more direct signals to him. Men, then, can no longer afford to make automatic assumptions on a woman's intentions simply because she is dressed to kill.

The ability to be able to change the style of the clothes to match the mood is a positive one, and gives a woman a greater flexibility in being able to express herself as a more all-rounded person rather than being fixed into a specific image. On the whole, a woman will probably be more clothes-conscious than her men friends, or her partner, but it is important for her to select her clothes to suit her colouring, height and size rather than try to emulate a particular style simply because it is fashionable.

A woman's size is not a barrier to her looking good if she takes the time to pick the clothes which flatter her particular body shape. She should forget about trying to copy any top-model look that happens to be in vogue. Feeling comfortable in what she wears is the most powerful way for a woman to be attractive, and

Power Play

▲ *This is a style of suit that means business. Sex is definitely secondary to ambition. However, there are enough feminine touches – the open neck and length of skirt – to show that the wearer has not sublimated her sexuality. She is saying, "I have got where I am because I am a woman – not in spite of my sex."*

most men respond to a woman who is relaxed and confident in herself, rather than only to the clothes that she happens to be wearing.

While revealing clothes can be fun to wear, and can certainly make a woman turn heads, sometimes the look can have a reverse effect on a man and actually scare him off. He might perceive the woman as a predatory man-hunter, and if he is not confident in his own sexuality, he may feel unable to cope with what he imagines will be her demands.

A Casual Approach

A woman may prefer to dress in such a way that she camouflages her more obvious sexual attributes, because she prefers men to be drawn to her because of her personality rather than her obvious feminine assets. She may prefer to wear comfortable clothes, like a shirt and jeans, that do not reveal too much of the shape of her body. In doing so, she feels more able to relate to men on an easy, equal and friendly basis rather than an immediately sexual one. This does not mean that she has switched off her sexual signals, but she is drawing attention to herself as a complete person with a mind and personality, as well as a feminine body.

Dressed to Impress

A man's clothes are likely to reflect his financial status and the power he commands as much as his sexual availability. A business suit, like a uniform, can indicate dominance and assertiveness and so conveys an air of

Easy Does It

▶ *In tight white jeans and denim top, open at the neck, this woman can present herself as undeniably feminine but is making it clear she is meeting the man on equal terms. Any relationship must be serious and include an appreciation of her as a person, not just a sex object.*

confidence and achievement. For some women, this aura of power is very sexually attractive, particularly if they seek a partner with whom they will feel secure and who is a successful and reliable provider. So a well-cut suit from a famed fashion designer, suggesting financial security and career success, could have definite appeal to these women. Even a man's casual clothes will often have an expensive branded trademark if he likes to dress to impress.

When a man is feeling sexually confident his clothes are likely to reflect the fact. Most men who keep themselves fit look good in jeans and T-shirts and although this is a common masculine attire, it is usually very attractive to women. Many find that the sight of well-

shaped buttocks, accentuated by the cut of a tight pair of jeans, is an extremely powerful turn-on. Men, like women, have increasingly broken the gender mould when it has come to dress, and a lot of men like to experiment with softer textures such as silk shirts, and brighter colours, moving away from the more traditional choice of dull grey and blue. This gives them the opportunity to express the more flamboyant, artistic or sensitive sides of their nature.

Both men and women dress to please and attract the opposite sex, but there is far greater freedom of expression nowadays for them to explore and project their own personality through what they wear without being inhibited by the constraints of gender conditioning.

Under Your Clothes

The choice of underwear a woman picks to put on before going out on a social or business engagement can make a major difference to the way she feels about herself. What items of clothing she has next to her skin, and that only she knows she is wearing, can do much to enhance her confidence and sense of attractiveness.

The colours can also affect her own mood, and definitely those of a lover if he sees her when she gets undressed. For instance, a red bra-

Frankly Scarlet
▼ *Sexy red underwear makes an unmistakably bold statement about you. It says you know what you want and nothing is going to stand in your way.*

and-panty combination can send a passionate message. In fact, for an overtly sexual statement you can't beat scarlet. It states that the woman is sexually confident and that she knows what she wants and plans to get it.

Black lacy underwear makes a sophisticated but feminine statement, and is flattering to any body shape. It is sultry and sexy while being practical, and shows the woman feels confident and in control. Sexy silk underwear in virginal white creates a wonderful contrast when worn under a smart but severe business suit. The soft material on the skin will feel very sensual and feminine. Silk underwear, in particular, is so smooth and teasingly flimsy that it gives a woman the daring impression that she is wearing nothing at all.

In contrast, sporty underwear that is comfortable and supportive helps a woman feel relaxed, knowing she can move easily and that her body looks and feels firm and secure.

Lacy Days
▲ Silky virginal white underwear will make you feel sexy and special – no matter what the day holds in store.

Nice and Easy
▶ Sporty and comfortable, this combination is not designed just for exercising to keep trim: it can make you feel relaxed and well supported under leisure clothes.

Body Language

According to psychologists, up to two-thirds of communication between humans is non-verbal. The way you sit or stand and the gestures you make broadcast a powerful message to the people you meet. While some of these signals may be given consciously, most body language is involuntary, either instinctive behaviour, or unconsciously learned through watching others. Even if you try to hide it, this secret code can reveal the way you truly feel. Understanding these subtle signs can indicate whether the person you feel drawn to is going to reject your overtures – or already feels the same way about you.

Our innermost thoughts trigger chemical and emotional changes in the body and we respond on a physical level by unconsciously altering our posture, expression and mannerisms. These responses may be subtle movements of the eyes and mouth, or more obvious statements, such as the way we fold our arms. Individually the signals may not amount to very much, but they all represent clues, like pieces in a jigsaw, that can fit together to reveal a picture of our true feelings.

Our body language is most expressive when we are with a member of the opposite sex. Men and women may not always be conscious of their feelings, but if they are genuinely attracted to another person, their bodies will broadcast the message loud and clear. Some responses are due to the fact that sexual attraction causes the body to release chemicals such as adrenaline, the "fight or flight" hormone, which causes the heart and breathing rate to quicken and so prepares a person for sudden hectic physical activity.

This leads to feelings of tension and restlessness, makes the mouth go dry and produces other signs associated with nervousness and embarrassment, such as a flushed face and sweating. These reactions are impossible to suppress.

Other human actions have their origins in evolutionary history. When birds follow a pattern of behaviour designed to attract a mate it is called a courtship display. We can see echoes of this avian mating ritual – the brightly coloured plumage, distinctive head actions, and changes in movement – in the behaviour of humans as they try to find a partner.

Yet the human mating game is far more sophisticated than that in the animal world, and as society becomes more complex, so does non-verbal communication. Body language now must cope with the subtle interplay of relationships between busy working men and women, both in their social lives and while pursuing demanding careers. As a result, the messages of body language are becoming increasingly difficult to decipher – and therefore more open to misinterpretation.

Confused Signals

Women complain that men often misread their signs. One reason for this may be that much of a woman's body language is concerned with creating a good impression generally,

Negative Signals

▲ *These body postures signal protection and defence. The arms are folded, closing off the emotional centres – the heart and belly – there is a distance between the couple, their eyes are averted and they are wearing bored expressions. There is no interest, and no chemistry.*

Opening Up

▲ *The body language here is starting to convey availability. Their bodies are leaning towards one another, and their arms and legs are in a more open posture, showing they are beginning to feel sexually at ease. A knee is extended to make that initial, exploratory touch.*

Making Contact

▲ *Their bodies are now getting energized as they feel safe enough in each other's company to really open up. They are smiling and making eye contact, his arm is on the back of the chair, ready to enfold her, and her hand is resting lightly on his knee.*

perhaps to a client, or business colleague, or to male and female acquaintances. In crowded work or social situations it may not even be clear who, if anyone, has caught the woman's interest, or she may give conflicting signals because she is unsure of herself or has other things on her mind. Her signals may not even be aimed at a single individual.

A woman who is unsure about the response she will get may look at everyone else in the room rather than the man she is attracted to, apart from an occasional glance. This is a signal that men often misread as indicating a lack of interest.

Differences in background can also lead to confusion. For example, a woman raised in an overly protective environment, or one where contact with males has been limited, may give out seemingly provocative signals when talking to men. She might be shocked to discover her behaviour was seen as a sexual invitation. On the other hand, the signals given out by a woman who is well used to male attention may be too discreet. Careful to avoid giving a false impression, her subtle signals might appear remote or even unfriendly.

A woman's natural fluency in body language means she can often spot when another female is attracted to a man before he can. He may even be unaware of being the focus of a female's attention, in the office or at a party, for example, until his partner points it out to him.

Men, too, must be careful about the signals they broadcast. As women tend to use delicate non-verbal cues with members of their sex, they can mistakenly believe that men are equally subtle and so get a false impression. What seems to be a brush-off may simply be a sign that a man is preoccupied with his thoughts.

Alternatively, a man may be thought to be showing genuine interest in a woman when, in fact, he is just being friendly, or going through the motions of flirting without any real intention of taking it further. To avoid such misunderstandings men and women must make an effort to decode the signals and so discover how the opposite sex really feels about them.

Complete rejection is usually easy to comprehend, but there are other more subtle signals which may suggest doubt or shyness. So never try to read body language in isolation or be too quick to jump to conclusions. It is important to weigh up all the signals before making a judgement. A man might be indicating a lack of interest if he evades your eye while talking to you, or he may just be shy.

A slumped posture could be a sign of rejection or that a man is feeling depressed and is having difficulty shaking the mood off.

At times, what seems like rejection might actually indicate confusion. If a woman sends out conflicting signals, seemingly interested but also defensive, it might be because her body is saying one thing but her mind is over-riding it. Such a situation may arise when a woman is in a long-term relationship with one man but is strongly attracted to another. She may be playing for time because she is not yet ready to reveal how she truly feels.

If your instinct tells you that a man is attracted to you, but he is not responding, there may be reasons for his negative body language. He may be recovering from a relationship in which he was badly hurt and so is wary of getting involved again too soon. He may already be in a relationship and so unable to show his feelings openly, or he may be incapable of making a commitment. It may even be that he considers you to be totally unattainable, even though he desires you.

Negative Signals

A round-shouldered stance, whether seated or standing, indicates that a man or woman is not feeling at ease. This message is often reinforced by a typical protective posture – arms folded defensively, knees held tightly together and legs or ankles crossed – in a subconscious desire to guard vulnerable parts of the body.

Sometimes a woman will sit or stand with her legs tightly entwined, with one foot locked behind the calf of the other leg, and she may place her hands protectively in her lap, unconsciously indicating that her genital area is off limits.

A man may signal rejection by turning right away from the other person, but in social situations it is usually only the lower half of the body that indicates the true state of affairs. For example, a man's head and torso are turned towards the woman and he appears to be concentrating on what she says, but his legs and feet point towards the exit door, indicating where his thoughts are leading him.

Men and women also use eye language to indicate rejection. These messages, known as "cut-off signals", indicate the desire to withdraw from a situation through lack of interest, or shyness. A woman will often glance round the room, as if

Getting Physical
▲ *His arm is around her shoulder and they are holding hands. The body language here is communicating intense interest and intimacy, mixed with tension, as their attraction to each other increases.*

calling out for someone to rescue her. It is an unspoken plea to be taken away from her companion, or for others to join the group, and so diffuse the situation.

Men and women may indicate stress through rapid blinking, or a blink that lasts longer than normal. They may also signal their unease by glancing rapidly to and fro, as if looking for someone, unable to settle their gaze on you.

Our social conditioning makes it difficult to be deliberately rude to people we meet, no matter how much we may dislike them. To avoid causing insult we are sometimes forced into telling white lies. This causes a conflict between what we say and how we feel, which is reflected in our body language. Small children automatically put a hand to their mouths when they tell a lie. In adults the gesture is more subtle. A person who is being evasive will often rub his nose, or hold a hand up to his cheek in a unconscious attempt to hide the falsehood.

If a man stands with his arms crossed and his thumbs pointing upwards he is communicating that someone is getting too close for comfort and is invading his body space. A similar defensive gesture is to sit with one arm placed across the body at waist level.

Accentuate The Positive

While body language is mostly involuntary, simple changes may improve the way you appear to others. If you are nervous or insecure you may give out negative signals, such as folding your arms, even when you want to be friendly. There are positive steps you can take to make yourself more inviting to other people, particularly members of the opposite sex.

It is vital to relax, particularly when meeting a man or woman for the first time. When you are tense your muscles tend to stiffen and this limits your repertoire of facial expressions and makes your movements seem jerky, awkward and ungraceful. It also makes you seem much older. You can reduce the tension in work or social situations, for example, by learning a relaxation technique such as deep, regular breathing whenever you feel nervous.

A natural smile, on the other hand, relaxes the facial muscles and has an instant effect on those around you, immediately putting them at

their ease. If the smile is genuine, a small group of facial muscles will make the skin form characteristic little crinkles around the eyes. These muscles are impossible to control consciously. In contrast, a false smile looks stiff and lasts longer than is natural.

It is also important to adopt an erect posture. Sitting or standing in a slumped, round-shouldered way creates a negative impression. For women in particular, it tends to be seen as a defensive posture that suggests you have put up barriers and are not inviting anyone to take the trouble to get to know you. Try to adopt a more open posture and you will seem more approachable.

A man should aim to hold the woman's gaze directly, without furtively glancing away, even if he is feeling nervous. Otherwise he can appear rather shifty. His gaze should be friendly, rather than deeply penetrating, which can appear fierce. An open, steady look that is softened with a smile can work wonders in smoothing the way to an introduction.

A major turn-off is a look that seems to linger over a woman's body, studying every curve. A man's urge to look at a woman's body is

natural, but he should do it in a respectful and appreciative way otherwise she will feel as if she is under a microscope.

The man who is most popular with the opposite sex is the one who makes each woman he talks to seem special by concentrating his gaze exclusively on her, without surreptitiously glancing at other females.

Relaying Availability

Men have a more limited non-verbal vocabulary than women when it comes to signalling interest in the opposite sex. Men often think they are making the opening moves in the mating game and so have less need of subtlety. In fact, it is a woman's more expressive body language that encourages the man she has chosen

Basic Attraction

▼ *The sexual signals are clear as they lean towards each other. His legs are wide apart, exposing his genital area. Her back is arched and her bottom is pushed out – it is a perfect example of primate sexual posturing.*

to make that first approach. Females have such a wide range of body postures, movements, and actions in their sexual armoury that males are often powerless to resist.

The way that males and females signal their availability is – initially – very similar in both sexes. When men and woman feel strongly attracted to someone they have seen for the first time, in the office or at a party, for example, the first sign is usually a change of posture. They will immediately sit or stand much straighter,

Mirror Images

Psychologists say that an important sign of whether a couple are forming a rapport is a type of behaviour called "mirroring". Here the man and woman unconsciously copy each other's actions or posture. For example, at a party if two people are sitting on a sofa deeply engrossed in conversation, the man may turn sideways and lean towards the woman, perhaps resting an arm on the sofa back. Almost immediately, this action is likely to be copied by the woman. If the woman crosses her legs the man will cross his too, or they will both raise their wine glasses and take a sip of their drinks at the same time. To observers these copy-cat actions will seem like mirror images.

Power Games

◀ *At first glance this couple look as if they are getting on well, but the pose is quite defensive. The woman is presenting herself, with her chest thrust forward, but her pulled-back pelvis indicates a withholding of her sexual energy. He is the opposite. His pelvis is forward, indicating sexual willingness, but his chest is pulled back and his arms are folded, suggesting emotional withholding. This is a classic "here I am but you can't have me" posture. They are playing power games as each suspects the other of wanting something that they are not willing to give in return.*

Little Girl Lost

She plays helpless and vulnerable, her defenceless posture signalling "I need to be rescued". He plays the macho super-hero, with puffed up chest, always in control, coming to her rescue. She fits right into his ego pattern, but no doubt has an agenda of her own.

which has the effect of making their tummy and neck muscles tighter and flatter, thereby giving a taller, leaner and more youthful outline.

A woman may arch her back so that her breasts are pushed out. She will often tilt her head back or to the side, exposing her sexually sensitive neck and making it seem longer and more elegant – a universal symbol of beauty. Preening actions, such as smoothing the dress down and patting the hair, are typical gestures at this stage, and, if walking, the

sway of the hips may become more exaggerated. If a woman is holding an object such as a wine glass, or cigarette lighter she may begin to stroke it rather suggestively while she looks at the man who has caught her interest.

A man may push his shoulders back and thrust his chest out, too, making his shoulders seem much broader, and his torso more muscular. Some sexually aggressive males may stand with both hands arrogantly placed on the hips and the chin jutting forward. If they are fairly assured of success they may lounge back in the chair with their hands behind their head. These gestures are designed to enlarge the man's outline, so making him look bigger and more powerful, and to create an air of confidence.

If men and women are strongly attracted to each other they may stand with their legs wider apart than normal. In women this stance makes such a powerful sexual statement

that it is regularly used by fashion models to make clothes look sexier. A relaxed, open stance also makes a woman seem friendlier and more approachable, so inviting the man to make contact.

At a party, a woman may sway in time to the music and glance at the male of her choice, inviting him to suggest that they dance together. This can be such a subtle gesture that men often feel that they instigated the approach without any prompting from the woman.

Male body language tends to draw attention to the genital region as the most overtly sexual signal. For example, a man will often sit with his legs spread apart to display his crotch, or he will stand with his pelvis thrust forward. One or both thumbs may be hooked into his belt or the waistband of his trousers, with the fingers pointing downwards towards the genitals to give extra emphasis. This pose is particularly common among adolescent males who have not learned a more subtle approach. A less blatant way of indicating the genital area is to stand with one hand inside a trouser or jacket pocket.

A woman's eyes will open much wider, giving her a welcoming and yet rather vulnerable appearance. She will look for an early opportunity to move closer to the man, even if she is currently engaged, perhaps talking to a close friend or an important client. If this is not immediately possible she will often turn towards him slightly to reduce the distance between them. If he is close by, this may draw him into the group, so providing an opportunity to initiate a conversation.

She may glance over her shoulder, or lower her eyelids and glance sideways until the man notices, and then quickly look away. If a woman lacks self-confidence she may never look at the man directly but only give side-long glances. A more overtly sexual gesture is to toss her head, flicking the hair out of her face, or she may run her hands through her hair, or lift it up behind her head.

Close Contact

Another sign of sexual interest is that a woman's feet will be pointing towards the man, often with one foot extended. She may touch him or brush against him, and keep her hand in contact with his for an extended time, when accepting a glass of wine or a light for her cigarette, for example. She may even allow her breast to touch the man's arm, as if unaware of the contact, and keep it there for a few moments.

Sitting down, her body will be turned towards him, signalling her interest and excluding all others. A woman will often sit with one leg tucked under the other and the knee pointed towards the man, and she may slowly cross and uncross her legs, or squeeze them together, tensing her leg muscles.

The man's body will also point towards the woman who has taken his fancy. This may start with just one foot aimed towards her, while his head and body are still directed at the person he is talking to. However, he will begin to turn his head towards the woman, to draw her into the conversation.

As his confidence builds he will move more of his body round to face her directly and will hold the woman's gaze for slightly longer than would normally be the case. He may lean across the woman, or move

A Meeting of Equals

▲ *Both are meeting on equal terms. Their open, balanced bodies indicate a willingness to communicate, without defences or preconceived expectations.*

round to exclude other group members who may be competing with him for her attention.

Displacement Activity

The special chemicals released in the body by sexual attraction cause a form of fidgeting and restlessness that is known as "displacement activity". This is the body's way of dissipating the nervous tension we feel when aroused by a member of the opposite sex. A man may straighten his tie, smooth his hair, or tuck his shirt in tighter. He may play with cuff-links, or remove imaginary pieces of lint, or specks of dust from his clothes, or he may be keep putting his hands in his pockets and taking them out again. The tension will make his mouth go dry, so he will need to clear his throat and lick his lips, and may run a finger around his collar, which will seem to have grown uncomfortably tight.

Women also show this displacement activity, indicating that a powerful sexual urge is being suppressed. Typical signals include playing with her jewellery, or twirling a lock of hair round a finger. She may swallow more than usual and may even wrap her arms around herself in an embrace. Other signs of attraction include gently stroking the thigh, and sliding a foot in and out of her shoe, or letting the shoe dangle from the toes.

More subtle sexual signals come into play once a man and woman are close together. A very feminine gesture is to hold a drink or a cigarette, for example, with her wrists and palms turned upwards or towards the man. This is a gesture that few males perform, except those who unconsciously want to appear more feminine.

Her head may also be angled to one side in a pose indicating rapt attention to his conversation. When she is speaking her tone of voice will become softer and lower in pitch. A husky female voice is considered sexy because it emulates the breathless quality of a woman who is very sexually aroused.

A woman's facial expressions also become much more eloquent and intimate. Her smiles will be broader and more frequent, and she will be quick to laugh at the man's attempts at humour – whether she finds them amusing or not.

A woman's lips represent a powerful sexual symbol. Some researchers believe the female mouth gives secondary signals about her genital area. The pouting open-mouthed look made famous by sex symbols such as Marilyn Monroe, the use of bright red lipstick, and the way a woman moistens her lips with her tongue to make them glisten, all emulate the female genitals, which open, redden and become shiny with her natural lubrication when she is sexually aroused.

The Language of Eyes

The eyes also provide an important indicator of sexual attraction. When a man sees something pleasurable, such as a beautiful woman, his eyes will dilate – as they would if he

had walked into a dimly lit room. This is a purely automatic response and cannot be faked. A woman's eyes also dilate when she is attracted to a man –

a sign men look for instinctively. One reason that a candlelit meal has long been associated with romance is that low lighting makes the pupils dilate, suggesting sexual interest. The women of Renaissance Italy used an extract of the deadly nightshade flower to dilate their pupils artificially and so make them appear more alluring, hence the plant's other name – belladonna, or "beautiful lady".

A female's eye language is particularly expressive, perhaps because of the important role that eye contact plays in establishing a bond with new-born babies. When a woman is with a man she finds attractive her eyes will grow wider and she will raise her eyebrows, to give an open and attentive air. Initially, the woman will look at the man often, but for brief moments only. Later on, she will hold his gaze for longer periods of time, but will still occasionally lower her eyes, demurely, to avoid making herself seem too forward.

If the relationship develops, both the man and the woman will stare into each other's eyes for extended periods of time. This is the clearest sign of all that a sexual rapport has developed between them. It is as if they exist in their own little world, apparently unaware of anyone else in the room.

Touching Moment
◀ *A light touch on the arm acknowledges closeness but is not invasive. The gesture does not come from a loaded or defensive stance, so it leaves the other person room to respond.*

First Encounters

The first moments in a relationship are very important. You are both nervous, unsure of yourselves and of how the other will react, yet desperately eager to create the right impression. You are aware that there is something special between you – the butterflies in the pit of your stomach and the light-headed feeling confirm that. But you are also worried that a careless move or a thoughtless word can spoil the mood and cause irrevocable harm to this budding relationship. Fear not, you must seize the moment. Remember, "Faint heart never won fair lady" – or man.

How a man and woman interact when they meet for the first time can set the seal on a relationship, or may crush a fledgling romance before it can take flight. A certain gaucheness now is understandable and acceptable. A slip of the tongue, a clumsy action – like knocking over a wine glass, or tripping over your feet – is to be expected when you are nervous about the way you will appear.

You are both eager to seem attractive, informed, interesting and sexy, but try to keep control of yourself – and the situation – and not let your tongue run away with you. You are keen to create a good impression, but don't start babbling on about yourself and stop the other person from getting a word in. At best, this can make you seem rather self-obsessed and conceited and may even appear that you have no interest in him or her but are simply looking for an available audience.

To avoid creating this impression, you should take every opportunity to draw the other person into the conversation. If you have been talking about a movie you saw recently,

Magic First Moments
◀ *The meeting place for that special first date will be special wherever you choose. But make sure it is somewhere you can talk and really get to know each other. A simple walk in the park will give you the time and space you crave, without the fear of irritating interruptions.*

ask your companion what he or she likes to see. If you have a favourite sport or pastime, try to find out about the other person's interests.

This approach is particularly important if your companion seems tongue-tied, perhaps through shyness or because he or she is unsure of the situation and anxious not to make a wrong move. Try to find areas of shared interest and keep to those, avoiding controversial topics, or subjects that seem to bore or irritate the other person. This will help you to discover whether you are compatible and may build a springboard from which you can launch the next stage of the relationship.

The First Date

No matter how well this first interaction with your new companion has gone, the relationship can still be nipped in the bud unless one of you plucks up the courage to ask the other for a date. Traditionally the man has been expected to make this first move. But now that women want to become more assertive in a relationship, this rule need no longer apply. Indeed, many men would be extremely flattered to be asked out by a woman.

However, no matter how confident some women are about other aspects of their lives, they may be reluctant to initiate the first approach. In that case they should steer the conversation in such a way that the man is encouraged to suggest a date. For example, a woman might mention in passing that there is a movie she has been keen to see, or she could ask if he knows anything about a rather cute little restaurant that has just opened. Whoever makes the suggestion, the

Give the First Date a Chance

Avoid choosing a night-club or pop concert for the first occasion. The noise and the crowd will make it difficult for you to hear each other, let alone talk, and you will probably have learnt little more about each other by the end of the evening than you knew at the beginning.

If you choose a movie, allow plenty of time to chat beforehand and conclude the evening with a visit to a bar or a restaurant so you have another opportunity to get to know each other.

Remember, though, the most idyllic settings are usually the simplest. If you are in reach of the coast, there is nothing like walking along a sandy seashore, as the setting sun casts golden reflections in the sea, to create an atmosphere of enchantment in which a relationship can flourish.

You could take a stroll in the park together – when there is an autumnal carpet of russet leaves covering the ground, or as the first buds of spring are peeping into view. Whatever the season, it is up to you to create the magic mood to match the moment. If the love affair develops these early trysts will always have an important place in your memories.

venue should be chosen with care on this all-important first date. You are still in the process of finding out about each other and need to select somewhere that will let you relate in an intimate atmosphere that is free from distractions.

The First Touch

Now that you are sure there is a developing bond between you, try to open up and reveal something about yourself, your hopes and aspirations, as well as your likes and dislikes. But don't just communicate your feelings verbally. Body language continues to play an important part in the way a couple interact, even after the initial meeting.

On this first date, try to avoid creating barriers, such as placing a handbag or umbrella between you, or folding your arms across your chest. Walking with your hands behind your back can also be taken as a defensive posture – that you are withdrawing into yourself. People react differently when courting, according

to their personality type, perhaps appearing very restless or withdrawn. Watch out for signs of tension or anxiety in your companion, such as tightly crossed ankles, or fidgeting with jewellery or cutlery, and look for ways to put her or him at ease.

Public Gestures

A simple touch of the hand can be very comforting, if it is done lightly, in a non-threatening way. Allow your fingers to brush against his, or take her hand in yours and give it a little squeeze. But don't make a sudden grab for the other person's hand before they are ready or it can be viewed as a show of power rather than a sign of affection.

By holding hands as you walk along you are providing a clear sign of your feelings. Many men are reluctant to display such a simple show of affection in public, yet to women it can mean a great deal. Women have often said that it was when their partner first held their

Holding Hands
▲ *Don't just hold hands palm to palm in the conventional way – intertwine your fingers, or give the hand a little squeeze, and gently stroke the highly sensitive skin on the inside of the wrist. These actions carry powerfully charged messages that can increase the electricity of the moment.*

hand in public that they realized the depth of their love.

If, perhaps out of shyness, the man does not make this move, it gives the woman an opportunity to take the initiative. This touching gesture from her reveals her feelings for him and can give his confidence a tremendous boost.

A comforting, protective arm round her shoulder is a simple enough gesture, too, but says far more than words can ever do. But the timing has to be right – watch for an instinctive flinching or tensing up on her part to indicate you have moved too soon. If

you sense this, don't remove your arm too quickly as this will show you have noticed her reaction and may embarrass her. Instead, wait a few minutes to take your arm away and then try again when your instincts tell you the gesture will be appreciated. If the relationship develops as you hope, you will soon be moving onto one of the most significant aspects of a new romance – the first kiss.

Sealed With a Kiss
It is natural to be over-anxious about the first kiss. Advertisements on television and in the glossy magazines

are designed to make us feel insecure about the way we smell and taste to others. Provided you have followed the basic rules of oral hygiene you can rest assured that your companion will be feeling just as insecure, and with as little reason.

However, if you are going to have a meal it is a good idea to avoid foods with really pungent aromas, such as garlic or onions, unless you know your companion is going to be eating the same thing.

A really confident, extrovert male may throw his arm round a woman and kiss her passionately on their first date. But with most women this rather proprietorial gesture is likely to lead to embarrassment and even hostility. Her body language will indicate this. She will tense up and look away, while her hands remain at her side showing no sign of returning the gesture. A better approach is to kiss her gently on the cheek, perhaps accompanied by the lightest of touches on the arm or shoulder.

Once you detect that a rapport has developed between you, the time will come to show your affection with a kiss on the lips. Unless you are sure that your partner is in the grip of an all-conquering passion – and that you feel the same way – it is best to keep this first mouth-to-mouth kiss as light and affectionate as possible. Again, the man is usually expected to make the first move – although there is no law that says this has to be the case.

A man will be looking for a sign from his companion that his advances will not be rejected. As he slowly edges forward he will notice whether she stays in the same place, or edges back defensively, or whether she mirrors his movements and leans forward too. She may lift her face to meet his and purse her lips slightly. If a woman closes her eyes as she kisses a man she is showing a clear sign of trust and affection, but this may not come until much later in the relationship.

Kissing can remain friendly and affectionate like this, or it can build up to become passionate and arousing. It takes sensitivity to know when the change is appropriate. It is not a good idea to plant a wet slobbering kiss on the lips, or to stick your tongue in someone's mouth before there is a tacit invitation to do so. At the same time, too much hesitation and uncertainty can be equally off-putting.

If you are beginning to explore a sexual relationship with a new friend, let the kissing experience build up its own momentum. Try to stay relaxed so that your mouth and lips remain soft and yielding. That will help you to avoid the embarrassment of clashing teeth that so frequently occurs during the teenage days of early sexual exploration.

In many ways, the sexual kiss reflects the sexual act itself, because it involves a close and intimate exchange of physical contact, and in the case of deep kissing, a mixing of body fluids as the tongue enters the warm, moist mouth. The contact of

mouth, lips and tongue, all highly sensitive and erogenous areas, can be an initial and safe way to discover whether there is a sexual chemistry and compatibility between you.

It Starts With a Kiss

▼ *When two people become sexually attracted to each other, the first mouth-to-mouth kiss usually signifies the change in the relationship. Let your partner's response dictate whether the kiss remains a light contact of the lips, or a passionate embrace with urgent thrusting tongues exploring each other's mouths.*

The Art of Wooing

Buoyed up by the success of that first romantic meeting, you feel as though you are floating on air, and the signs are that your new friend feels the same. No matter how well that first date seemed to go, the start of a new relationship is a nerve-racking period filled with opportunities for mistakes and misunderstandings. At this critical juncture, your next steps may decide whether you will part merely as friends or whether the relationship will develop into a lasting love affair. If both sides are honest and say how they feel, there is more chance that the relationship will be successful.

This is an anxious time as you wonder whether the person you have fallen for also feels the same way about you and would welcome another meeting. Waiting for someone to telephone to arrange another date can be agonizing, so, if you have had a good time, pick up the telephone and tell her how much you enjoyed the evening.

Suggest a second date within the next few days to judge whether your feelings are reciprocated. If you get the brush-off you must be philosophical; there is no easy way to deal with disappointment other than to hope to meet someone else soon. But if your companion is keen to see you again give plenty of encouragement.

It is important to nurture the friendship by keeping in contact and setting regular dates to meet. Try to vary the venues and activities to keep the relationship fresh and alive. Look for shared interests and try to capitalize on them by arranging activities you can take part in together. For example, if you both enjoy jogging, or have just talked about starting an exercise programme, arrange regular running sessions together. If you both enjoy the movies, set aside one night a week to see the latest releases.

Even if your pastimes are very different, try to take an interest in the other person's pursuits. It won't hurt you to attend a classical music concert or a football game occasionally, and you may even enjoy it.

At the same time, try not to be over-enthusiastic. Give your new friend the space to continue with his or her own life and to maintain other friendships. This will avoid giving the

Keeping In Touch
◀ *If you have enjoyed the evening, say so. A call from you will dispel any nagging doubts she may have about the success of your first date and a call at other, unexpected, times will show you have been thinking of her.*

impression that you are trying to push the relationship on too quickly. If you spend time away from each other, it will ensure your days together are even more vibrant.

Keeping Romance Alive

Just because you are getting to know one another, don't take the relationship for granted and let the romance of those heady early days begin to slide. Look for ways to show your feelings, for example by giving a present when you next meet. This should be a simple token of affection and not an expensive gift loaded with expectation, as though you expect something in return. Flowers, especially red ones, the colour that more than any other signifies love, still represent one of the most romantic statements a man can make. A woman, too, should play her part in the art of wooing by presenting the man with little gifts, such as a bottle of his favourite wine. As well as being a touching gesture in itself, this shows she has taken the trouble to discover his tastes.

Showing consideration and an awareness of the other person's moods and feelings can also enhance the loving feelings between two people. For example, a simple gesture such as helping a woman on with her coat, or complimenting her on her hair or dress, shows you really care.

Notice that your friend is tired after a busy day at the office and suggest that you cancel the date you had planned that evening, or leave early, even though you may have been looking forward to it. Your companion will really appreciate the fact that you are so finely attuned to his or her emotional wavelength and are willing to put another's best interests before your own.

Shared Interests

▶ *Find an interest that you have in common, such as jogging, and make it a regular part of your weekly schedule. Finding a sport or pastime you can share is the quickest way to cement a friendship.*

Food of Love

Once the relationship is at a stage where you feel confident enough to do so, it is natural to want to invite your new friend to your home for a meal. A sultry candlelit dinner is still one of the most romantic settings for a couple during the early stages of a relationship. It provides just the right ambience to open up to your new friend.

This does not have to be an exclusively female gesture. Males are just as capable of preparing a meal and a woman will be enchanted by this sign of a man's thoughtfulness. Cook only what you can comfortably handle. If the menu is too elaborate you will be tired before the meal starts and are likely to be spending all your time fretting about the next course, rather than enjoying your friend's company. You may also feel resentful if he or she shows less appreciation for your efforts than you think you deserve.

The atmosphere, rather than the food, is the most alluring aspect of the dinner, so aim to set the right mood. Low lighting is important to create the feeling of closeness, so you can relax and reveal your innermost thoughts. But don't rely on candles alone for the lighting. If the room is too dark it can seem forbidding rather than comforting. The room should be pleasantly warm but not stifling, or you will both feel sleepy rather than

Language of Flowers

▼ *The simplest message often speaks volumes and a gift of flowers, whether as a large bouquet or a single red bloom, is unmistakable. It shows that you care about her, without hinting that you might expect something in return.*

romantic, so leave a window ajar to ensure there is adequate ventilation.

A vase of fragrant flowers adds a spring-like touch, and romantic music playing softly in the background will help enhance the mood, but make sure it is quiet enough for you to hear each other without raising your voices. Your aim is to create an island of intimacy, cut off from the cares of the outside world.

This is a time to talk and share and be as one with each other. How much of yourself you reveal in these intimate encounters is entirely up to you, but it is better to be as open as possible, rather than hold back and risk creating an emotional distance between you.

Expectations

This can be a crucial time in a relationship. The food, the wine, the warm, moodily lit romantic atmosphere, can make your dinner date seem the sexiest companion in the world. Once you have opened up to your "significant other" on an emotional level you will be better able to judge whether you want to take the relationship on to a more physical stage.

Whether that means passionate kissing and heavy petting, penetrative sex, or any of the sexual possibilities in between, this is a very personal decision that individuals must make themselves, according to their own moral codes and social mores.

The question of when to sleep together for the first time has always been fraught with ethical and practical worries. In the past, the main concern has been the fear of pregnancy. The greater availability of effective contraception has largely removed that fear for many couples

A Thoughtful Gift

▲ *A romantic gift should show some thought and consideration for the other person. A bottle of his favourite wine suggests that you have taken the trouble to discover his preferences.*

(although, on religious grounds, it may still not be an option for other people) but this concern has been replaced by the risk of HIV infection.

It is not unusual for some couples to have sex on the very first date, while others prefer to reserve sex until after marriage, or ensure that it is part of a clearly committed long-term relationship. For most modern couples, however, the change of pace from simple friendship to sexual intimacy is likely to occur at some point between these two extremes. It might be after a second or third date, or it may be that a couple will not feel they know each other well enough to take this step until several weeks or even months have elapsed.

However you feel about the issue, it is your decision and you should not feel pressurized into having sex before you are ready, nor should you coerce others to do so.

No matter how aroused you become, you will need to remain highly attuned to your partner's signals, ready to slow the tempo, or stop altogether, if there are any signs of nerves, or hesitation. A man, in particular, is making a very grave error if he assumes that his sexual technique is so irresistible he will be able to get a woman into a state of sexual arousal in the face of her obvious signs of reluctance.

A woman's right to say "no" to sexual intercourse must always be respected, regardless of whether a couple have had sex on previous

Candlelight Romance

▲ *A romantic meal can set the seal on a developing love affair. Bathed in the warm glow of candlelight you can lose yourselves in the magic of the moment and enjoy just being with your companion, free from the cares and distractions of the outside world.*

occasions, or have been enjoying a highly arousing session of kissing and petting, and no matter how passionate her sexual signals may have seemed beforehand.

Her cooling off need not imply that the woman is a "tease" or that she has suddenly lost interest in the man, merely that she is not in the mood or is not yet ready to let the relationship develop to that stage.

Just as men have always been expected to make the opening moves in a sexual encounter, a woman should also be free to take the initiative and invite the man to stay overnight if she chooses. And if the man declines, for whatever reason, or no reason at all, this should not be taken as a rejection or a lack of

sexual interest. It may simply be that he is not ready to make that commitment, or is tired, or has drunk a little to much alcohol, and is worried that his sexual performance will prove to be a disappointment to her.

A sensitive lover is one who can read his companion's mood and knows how far to go. Constant oblique references to sex, or overly passionate kisses when the other person is clearly not responding, are more likely to make them feel cold and resentful, rather than sexually aroused.

When two people are attuned to each other's needs and desires, eager to give pleasure as well as receive, and ready to consummate the relationship with a physical display of their love – the sky's the limit.

Chapter 5
Enhancing Sex

When a relationship has become established into a routine pattern it is all too easy for a couple to take each other for granted. Like putting on a comfy pair of slippers, you know exactly what to expect from each other. But this is also fraught with pitfalls because once you begin to feel that you know your partner inside out you can miss the signs that indicate when things are not well in a relationship. To avoid this you need to develop your communication skills so that you can stay attuned to your partner's innermost thoughts and desires. But in addition you need to find new ways to enhance your sexual relationship, to adapt to the changes that age and ill-health can make, to experiment with new approaches to your sexuality and sensuality, such as learning how to massage each other lovingly, or by playing games and exercises. Also, you can seek to enhance the spiritual dimension of your sexual relationship, learning to make love in a new and meditative way.

Communication Skills

Communication and listening skills are essential keys to unlock the tensions and problems which inevitably occur in any ongoing relationship. They enable you to verbalize those issues that are important to you, and help you to express your most vulnerable and emotive feelings, without descending into a tirade of blame and criticism that will only serve to alienate your partner.

Learning to listen carefully to your partner's thoughts, values, opinions and feelings without the need to become defensive, or argumentative ensures that open and honest communication continues between you. If both of you determine to practise the communication and listening skills described in this section whenever problems arise, you may be able to respond more positively to difficult situations. In this way you can support, understand and accommodate each other's needs and differing opinions.

No relationship is without its stresses and strains. In the beginning, when you first fall in love, the pull of your mutual attraction can mask aspects of your individuality and ego and also blind you to the truth about your partner's personality. Only when your relationship settles down do your personal views, values, needs and temperaments begin to emerge in detail. If you marry, or form a long-term relationship, create a home together, raise children and pursue demanding careers, inevitably these additional challenges will test your relationship in different ways. While you strive to make your relationship a secure and nurturing base from which you can both draw emotional and physical support, you must also constantly adapt and respond to life's ever-changing realities.

Everyone evolves in mind, body and spirit as they mature. No one can expect a partner to remain exactly the same as when they first met. Nor can you stop the process of change within your own life, and you may come to realize that the things which made you happy or content in earlier years may no longer bring you such fulfilment. As in any partnership, there will be a constant need for negotiation if you wish to navigate your relationship safely and successfully through the turbulent waters of life.

Areas of Conflict

There are countless situations in which the needs and boundaries of a relationship have to be carefully re-examined and re-defined. Small issues can build up into a major area of conflict if you fail to communicate your needs, or listen to one another.

For example, you might feel neglected by your husband because he watches football at the weekends, leaving you feeling aggrieved and abandoned. Perhaps your partner has forgotten your birthday, or a wedding anniversary, and you take that as a sign that he no longer cares about you. Maybe you feel your girlfriend criticizes and harasses you, especially at those times when you feel most under stress. Or she resents your friends, and that makes you feel she is trying to change you.

Issues can be intensely personal, such as the way you make love, whether you are honest with one another, the degree of intimacy you share, and whether you care enough about each other. Domestic problems can arise over the housework, parental responsibilities, and especially over the finances.

In almost every area of a relationship, some rules and boundaries need to be made to help it function well. Two mature adults should be able to make agreements which incorporate their mutual needs. Even so, those rules will be subject to change and re-negotiation as time goes by.

The Need to Stay Cool
◀ *Avoid accusatory statements, harsh words and criticism. Be aware of body language – hardening your eyes and mouth or pointing your finger will make him defensive.*

Words You'll Regret

▲ *Bombarding each other with personal insults, shouting or talking louder than the other person, or aggressive words and actions will alienate you from each other, ensuring neither of you has a chance to communicate or even be heard above the din. Words spoken in the heat of the moment are often greatly regretted once your tempers have had a chance to cool down.*

Attacking the Ego

▲ *Don't undermine your partner's self-esteem in order to accentuate your point of view. It will only make her angry or hurt. Overwhelmed by these feelings, she is totally incapable of hearing your side of the story. Her body language may demonstrate that she is virtually cutting off all her points of access to you, by covering her face, ears, eyes and mouth.*

Signs of Stalemate

▲ *The body language here clearly indicates that both partners are saying "back-off". If you have failed to communicate and listen carefully, then you are probably going to reach a stalemate situation where nothing more is going to be resolved. Things may carry on relatively normally for a while, but both of you have become even more entrenched in your own points of view. Sooner or later the attack will begin again.*

Listen Without Judgement

▲ *Instead of using verbal tactics, take it in turns to discuss your feelings and needs and state clearly what is bothering you about a certain situation. Take responsibility for how you feel, using "I" rather than the accusatory "You". Keep eye-contact and let your bodies be open and undefended towards each other, and remember to breathe deeply so you stay relaxed. Listen carefully to what your partner has to say to you, avoiding judgement or criticism.*

Taking Responsibility

Words of war will never heal a relationship or help you and your partner to find a solution to troublesome issues. In good communication, you need to take responsibility for your own feelings instead of blaming your partner for your emotional state. Accusation will force him or her into the mode of protection and the need to block your words, either by retaliating with a damaging counter-attack or by withdrawing.

Comparing your partner negatively or with derision to someone else is demeaning to that person, and can only result in more anger or bad feelings. Insulting your partner's family, friends or beliefs can deeply hurt his or her feelings and cause lasting damage to a relationship.

Manipulation may work in your favour temporarily, but your partner will know he has been duped. If you threaten your partner, you may gain a tentative victory, but revenge is likely to be in store. Making your mate feel guilty about who he is will guarantee defensive behaviour, and criticism can only serve to lower your lover's self-esteem.

Stubbornness demonstrates an unwillingness to work on a solution and an entrenched point of view. If you placate your partner, you are dismissing her needs and avoiding the real nature of the issue, and withdrawal is the ultimate weapon of power because your absence leaves the other person feeling helpless.

What you say is one thing, and how you say it is another. Shouting and raising your voice "deafens" your partner, and continually repeating yourself, nagging, complaining or whining is guaranteed to make your partner react in a negative way.

Listening Well

How you listen to your partner complements your communication skills. You can hear the words, but still not listen to their content. You can make your own judgements about what your partner is saying, while failing to comprehend what she is really trying to get across.

Listening to someone with an armoured or defended attitude which says "Here we go again" indicates that you are unwilling to be receptive. Imagining that you know what

is best for your partner and your relationship means that you are unable to consider the other person's point of view. Thinking up a retaliatory statement while your partner is speaking to you renders you incapable of listening at all. Tuning-out is the aural version of physical withdrawal – you are not going to hear what your partner is saying if you have one eye on the television and the other on your newspaper.

All of the above are typical examples of relating patterns which any of us may employ when real communication breaks down. Instead, we may revert to our "parental voices" blaming and punishing. If we are on the receiving end of this critical tirade, the "child" within us is provoked and it is inevitable that the reaction that ensues will be petulant, hysterical, sullen, angry or argumentative.

Communication and Listening Exercise

Communication between two people who love each other should never become a power struggle, or a battle to win at all costs. It should be a

Repeat to Show You Hear

◀ *Reflect back to your partner what you think you have heard her say so she can correct any misunderstandings that may have occurred. The fact that you have absorbed her words and are able to feed them back to her so succinctly will restore her confidence in the relationship because she will feel you have listened carefully to her.*

Listen to the Other Side

◀ *Once you have expressed your needs and feelings and felt that your partner has fully understood them, allow him the chance to respond in a similar way. Now it is your turn to listen carefully to his point of view. If he doesn't think he is going to be criticized or judged, he may be able to reveal aspects of himself that he has previously felt unable to show. Focus carefully on what he has to say, nodding or smiling to show you have grasped its content. Even if you do not share his opinion, let him express it.*

Tackling the Issues

▼ *The communication exercise will enable both of you to move positively towards solving a tricky dilemma because you will have gained an understanding of each other's feelings and needs. This will provide you with the useful tools with which to tackle the issues involved, and hopefully find a suitable solution.*

mutual search to try to understand and support each other, respectful of the needs of both the individual and the relationship. It takes courage to talk about your feelings honestly and to take responsibility for them, and diligent awareness to locate the true source of your emotions and unhappiness. It needs respect and empathy to listen carefully to what your partner is saying without immediately feeling threatened, or needing to defend your corner.

If you are experiencing communication problems within your relationship, you can try the following exercise which allows you to explain your needs and opinions clearly, and to listen empathically to your partner's truth. At first the exercise may seem awkward and too formal but this is because it is a new way of sharing with each other.

When an important issue is at stake, or whenever you are feeling hurt about something within the relationship, make an appointment with each other specifically to sit and talk it over. Resolve to do this calmly and without recrimination, and try to enter this communication exercise with an open heart and mind. Relax your body and breathe deeply so you release pent-up tensions before you begin.

Sit opposite your partner so you can have eye-to-eye contact. You may find it more comfortable to have a table between you which you can consider as a neutral arena. Uncross your arms and legs so your body language is not defended, avoid using your eyes to intensify your words, or gritting your teeth, or tightening your jaw, and do not point your finger accusingly at your partner.

One partner takes five minutes to speak while the other's task is simply

Sharing the Workload

▲ *When both partners are working outside the home, household tasks need to be shared. How you negotiate that division of labour should take into consideration your needs and preferences, the time that either of you expect to put into the housework, and when any particular task should be done. There should be flexibility in the arrangement, so, for example, if your partner is working late, you may offer to cook the dinner – even if it isn't your turn.*

to listen. If you are the speaking partner, state clearly what your feelings are and what is bothering you. However, take responsibility for those feelings. Avoid phrases like: "You don't love or care about me any more. You are so selfish around the house and you never do your share of the chores. You make me feel like I'm the servant here."

Instead, phrase this in a different way, such as: "I realize that over the last weeks I have been getting very angry and snappy towards you. I am finding my work very stressful at the moment, so when I come home, I do not feel able to cope with the cooking

and housework alone. Recently, I have been doing most of the tasks in the evenings. What I would like is for us to draw up a new agreement on how we can share the jobs."

In this way, you have spelt out your needs clearly. You have identified your emotions and put them in a context. In addition, you have explained, without accusation, why you need extra support at this time, and you have offered a framework for a solution.

As the listening partner, you do not interrupt or defend yourself, and this is made easier by the fact that you are not being blamed for the situation. You can show your partner that you are listening to her empathically by leaning towards her as she speaks, or nodding your head to show you are assimilating her words.

At the end of the five minutes, sum up for her what you believe you have heard her say. In this way you reflect back to her the content of her communication, and by repeating it, you absorb the information better. Your feedback enables her to correct any misunderstandings you may have gained as to what she actually said and it assures her that you have been actively listening.

Swapping Roles

Now it is the listening partner's turn to speak. If you do not feel ridiculed or criticized, you have a better chance of communicating your own version of the situation. In the past you may have retorted with something like: "You never stop nagging. Sometimes your complaining makes me so sick that I want to walk out. Anyway, the house looks perfectly fine to me – the problem is that you are neurotic". This reply is a defensive attack which

◀ *Household jobs do not have to be turned into chores, they can be a great opportunity for you to spend some time together, joking and chatting over the day's events. After dinner, rather than one partner being relegated to the kitchen while the other person goes to another room, why not share the washing-up tasks? That way, you can catch up on the gossip, and create extra time for relaxing together.*

manages to combine an accusation, a threat, a denial and an insult all in one delivery!

During this exercise, you have more chance to respond rather than to react in the manner above. You might tell her instead: "I've also had a lot of pressure at work recently, and when I come home, my immediate need is to take time to unwind. The difficulty between us seems to be that you like to get things done straight away while I prefer to do them later, or at the weekends. What usually happens is that you go straight ahead with the chores, and I usually skulk off feeling guilty. I am very willing to do my half of the work, but my main priority is that we make more time to relax and enjoy each other's company in the evenings."

If you are now the listening partner, you should summarize and reflect back what your partner has just told you and allow him to correct you if you have misheard any of the content of his communication. If you need more time to continue your reciprocal communication exercise, then you can use its structure again. If you were to use the above example of the exercise, it would have enabled you to refrain from blame and criticism, while stating clearly your paramount needs.

You have established a framework in that you both agree that the housework needs to be done and the chores shared, but you now need to discuss how the jobs can be better divided and when is the best time to do them. You will need to negotiate a solution which encompasses the needs and wishes of both of you, but that will be far easier to do if neither of you feels angry or in the wrong.

Unless relationship issues are dealt with as they arise, their undercurrents are likely to affect other aspects of your lives. Sexual disharmony or reduced intimacy and affection can often be a reflection of other unresolved issues, rather than being directly related to sexual problems. Good communication and listening skills are as important to the health, harmony and growth of your relationship as is the happiness of your sex life.

Catharsis

Pent-up feelings of anger and frustration can become locked in your body's musculature, making you feel tense and irritable, and more inclined to provoke arguments in the home. Sometimes the cause of these feelings is not directly related to anything that has happened between you and your partner, but your charged emotions spill out and you react negatively to the slightest comment. Perhaps you are under stress at work, or you have been angered or disappointed by a certain event, or maybe there are issues in your relationship that you are too wound up about to discuss rationally.

One way of helping to discharge this emotion in a safe way, without hurting or blaming any one else, is by catharsis. By acting out and giving vent to your feelings when you are alone, you can release your intense emotions.

Beating the cushions is a method that is sometimes used in therapy sessions, enabling clients to express their anger in a non-harmful way. You can do this in the privacy of your home, too, though it would be better to wait until you are alone. You can shout and yell at the same time, if you can do so without disturbing the neighbours.

Let rip for up to ten minutes, giving yourself permission to discharge your rage into the cushions by beating your fists against them. By allowing yourself to feel and express your anger without judgement, it may transform itself into a wave of non-emotive energy which will leave you feeling full of vitality as your tension blocks are released.

Sometimes, sadness lies behind anger and you may get in touch with your more vulnerable feelings. If the anger turns into tears, then hug the pillow to your body, and allow yourself to cry until you feel a release from your pain. When you have experienced your catharsis, rest for at least five minutes, and breathe deeply so your whole body relaxes.

If this technique is suitable to you, then use it at times when you feel your body racked with emotion but are unable to express your feelings adequately in words. This way no one else gets hurt, and you may find it a great relief.

If you cannot imagine yourself undergoing catharsis, another good way to release pent-up frustration is through strenuous physical activity, such as running, brisk walking or dancing. Try to breathe deeply and move your body freely in order to discharge all your tensions and regain a sense of equilibrium.

Being Vulnerable

No matter how mature and responsible we have become as adults, a part of us remains child-like, retaining the vulnerable and playful elements of

Expressing the Anger
▲ Build a pile of cushions in front of you on a supportive base such as the mattress on your bed. Make fists and begin to pound the cushions. At first you may feel self-conscious and resistant to expressing your anger in this physical way. Get in touch with your emotions and allow them to gather momentum and express themselves through your body. Release the tension from your body.

Releasing the Tension
▲ If you feel able to shout and yell without disturbing other people, then do so and this will help you clear the emotional tension that has been "choking" you. You can even say all the nasty things you have been carrying in your mind and let them evaporate into thin air. This will help you to dispel your more negative thoughts so that later you can approach your problems more calmly.

The Inner Child
▼ Even as an adult there are times when you will need to be comforted and supported by your mate. A partner who is able to respond to your "inner child", and is not afraid of it, is secure in himself and in touch with his own sensitive side.

our nature. If you accept that part of yourself, and learn to love your "inner child", it will help make you a more balanced person and better able to respond to those aspects in your partner. The inner child is the part of your personality that is magical and inquisitive, but that also feels insecure and is easily hurt. It is the part of you that sometimes needs nourishment, comfort and reassurance.

In an adult relationship, there will be times when the "child" within one partner will meet the "parent" within the other. A balanced relationship is one in which these roles can be shared, so that you are able to respond to each other appropriately in times of need.

Long-Term Relationships

Your sexual relationship may improve with time as you and your partner become increasingly compatible on an emotional and physical level. As intimacy grows between you, and the relationship becomes stable, you may be better able to relax together in every way. In these circumstances, your sexual relationship can mature with age like a vintage wine.

Many women are only able to open up sexually once they feel emotionally secure, finally reaching their true orgasmic potential when they trust that they are truly loved. For some men, the early stages of a relationship can be fraught with tension, particularly the pressure to perform well in bed. They may be so nervous and excited in the early stages of a relationship that they engage in intercourse with undue haste and ejaculate prematurely. Only when they have relaxed into a sexual relationship can they allow the more sensual side of their nature to shine through in their lovemaking.

Time and familiarity will allow you and your partner to know each other's arousal responses, to tune in to your mutual sexual needs, and to feel increasingly comfortable with your own and each other's bodies. As sex is an expression of caring as well as desire, your lasting and loving relationship can, by its very nature, enrich your sexual exchange.

Knowing and trusting each other well gives you the opportunity to explore new avenues within your sexual preferences. The safety of the relationship may allow you to reveal and act out your sexual fantasies and this can add an extra erotic input into your conjugal activities.

Changing Patterns

If you are in a long-term relationship, your sexuality may pass through many phases, and it would be highly unusual if it never changed in content or style from your early days of

A Deepening Sexuality

▲ Intimacy, deepening companionship, and knowledge of each other's bodies and physical responses can enhance your sex life in a long-term relationship. As both of you relax deeply into your sexuality, it can become more expansive, creative and loving.

Spicing Up Your Love Life

▶ Confidence in the relationship, and trust with each other, may inspire you to reveal and experiment with some of your more playful sexual fantasies. This is also a good way to pep up your sex life when things have become dull and routine. A little kitchen erotica may convince him that there is more on the menu than just supper!

romance. For the reasons mentioned above, it can steadily improve, and it may enhance in quality if not in quantity. However, there may come a time when the frequency of your sexual activity declines after you have lived together for more than a few years.

Seeing each other every day, and concerning yourselves with the other important demands in your lives, you may no longer have the energy, wish, or need to make love with the same intensity as when you first met. Quite naturally, like any two people who begin to build a home together and improve on their careers, or decide to start a family, you may focus your attention on other matters of mutual and personal concern.

The passion which drew you together and ignited the flame of your love is unlikely to sustain itself with the same degree of desire throughout the duration of your long-term relationship. The familiarity which makes your partnership so comfortable and supportive can be the very thing which erases the excitement of the earlier days, when just the sight of each other would be sufficient to arouse you.

Seeing your lover every day, and sharing the hard times as well as the good, may create a supportive and nurturing relationship, but does not necessarily arouse the libido to the same extent as before.

Often, these changing patterns of sexual behaviour will settle into an easy and compatible rhythm which happily satisfies you both. There will be times when your sexual interest rises, and periods when it subsides, and this will largely be affected by outside pressures, such as stress, the needs of your children, the demands of your work, and the general accord between you both in other areas of your lives.

Differing Sexual Needs

Problems may occur in an established partnership, however, if you and your mate develop very different patterns of sexual need. One of you

A New Kind of Intimacy

▶ *It is perfectly normal for the frequency of sexual activity to subside after some years in an established relationship as passion gives way to closeness and intimacy of a different nature. This can be a mutually satisfying situation if there is no great disparity in your sexual needs. Just being together, relaxed and aware of each other, while quietly involved in your own activities, can be a very nourishing experience in itself.*

Lovers and Friends

▶ *One of the most wonderful aspects of a long-term relationship is that it can deepen your friendship with each other. Once you know that you can see each other as much as you like, the sexual pressure begins to subside and you can explore many different avenues of pleasure and leisure. You can learn new pursuits, pastimes and games to enjoy and just keeping each other company will be rewarding and relaxing.*

may lose interest in sex altogether, or be content with occasional sexual episodes. What one of you might regard as an adequate level of love-making might be vastly different from the other's expectations.

There is no rule that dictates how often a couple should make love. You may feel deprived if you are not having sex every day, whereas your partner may think that three times a week is a happy routine. The disparity could be even greater, with one of you believing that once a week is sufficient for your needs while the other is rarely interested in making love more than once a month.

One of you might even lose interest in sex altogether, especially when

you have been together for a number of years, or following illness, childbirth, the loss of a parent, or promotion to a more stressful job. The emerging differences in sexual needs can create a severe problem if you do not look at the issues, adapt to the changes, and reach a mutually satisfying arrangement that suits your varying levels of libido.

The one who is more deprived can feel aggrieved, and personally rejected. If you are in this position, you may begin to put pressure on your partner, berating the person you love, and you may feel demeaned by your unsatisfied sexual needs.

If you are the one who has lost interest in sex, you may resent your partner's desires, and even begin to feel that he or she is making unreasonable demands on your time and intimacy. A situation like this, if it is allowed to develop unchecked, becomes a vicious cycle. One of you will become increasingly obsessed with the need for sex,

Rekindle the Flames of Passion

▼ *Make love in parts of the house other than the bedroom so that the change of setting inspires new and delightful ways of lovemaking. If you have one, light the fire in your living room hearth and abandon yourselves before its flames. By breaking old patterns of sexual behaviour, you can keep your relationship very alive.*

Dealing with Sexual Disparity

◄ *There are many reasons why you and your partner may have differing sexual needs. At various times, and for different reasons, a low libido can affect either one of you. If this continues, and is affecting the happiness of your relationship, you will need to explore the reasons and find some way to improve the situation.*

while the other may withdraw and become even less romantically inclined.

A couple may allow time to pass before realizing the extent of the problem or feeling sufficiently resolved to face up to its issues. This dilemma may be compounded by the difficulty of talking about sexual matters – a subject in which egos can so easily be bruised. Tact, diplomacy and negotiation, however, are needed to approach and address the subject. If you are facing this situation, you will need to develop your communication skills so that you can explore your varying sexual needs and

Seeking Spiritual Uplift

► *After a time, the passion and heat of sex may no longer enthral you. You may seek to change the quality of your lovemaking into something that is more sensual and increasingly spiritually and emotionally uplifting. If you are able to let go of the excitement of sex, and make love in a more meditative way, your intimacy and bonding will continue to flower.*

feelings. You may then discover the root cause of your differences and find new ways to resolve it.

Be Creative

One of the main causes for your sexual indifference may be that your love-life has become too routine. Flopping into bed after a busy day may not provide the ideal scene for an ardent encounter. Try to create new and exciting opportunities for lovemaking, away from the more predictable situations. Make love in the living room instead of the bedroom, or stay at a hotel for the weekend. The change of

Looking and Feeling Good

◀ *Familiarity in a relationship is no reason to lose interest in looking and feeling good about your body. The desire to remain attractive will continue to matter to your partner and will boost your own feelings of self-worth. When you plan a romantic evening in or out, first soak in a relaxing bath perfumed with aphrodisiac essential oils. Moisturize your skin so it is soft to the touch. Little efforts like this show you are not taking the relationship for granted.*

environment can make sex more adventurous and exciting.

Alter the timing of your sexual interludes, so you make love in the afternoon, morning or early evening before you get too tired. Bring a little spice and passion back into your love-life with the occasional "quickie" session of spontaneous sex to recapture the fervour of earlier years.

Sexual fantasies are an excellent aphrodisiac and you may like to explore together new and exciting variations of sexual behaviour. It is also possible that as your intimacy deepens in other aspects of your partnership, lusty sex is no longer appealing to you. In this case, why not try a different way of making love which is less orientated towards orgasm and performance and more focused on being meditative, sensual and calm.

When You Have Children

If the responsibility of childrearing has become the main focus of your relationship, seek a way to balance your love and caring so that your partner is equally included. It is easy to feel that, as parents, your sexual and emotional life must take second place to the needs of your children.

In the first months after the birth of a new baby, sheer exhaustion causes the libido to flag and this is a normal and usually temporary state of affairs. But if you start to perceive your partner or yourself only in terms of "mother" or "father", your sexual relationship may begin to suffer.

However, the strength of your family rests on the supportive and loving bond which exists between you as adults and, if this remains the primary relationship, you and your children will greatly benefit.

Try to create some time when you can be alone together, away from domestic demands. This may be difficult, especially when the children are young, but resolve to make it possible. Look for a reliable baby-sitter and give yourselves an evening off once in a while to go to the cinema, the theatre, a restaurant or just for a walk.

If you have a loving extended family, then as the children get older perhaps a relative could take care of them for the occasional weekend while you and your partner go away for a break. Adjustments like this in your relationship will help to keep your romantic feelings alive and vibrant.

Bathing and Bonding

▼ *Whether or not you have an active sex life at the moment, find ways to keep the sensuality alive in your relationship. Soaking together in a bath of aromatic oils provides delicious skin-to-skin contact. Massage and stroke each other's bodies; this tactile stimulation will leave you feeling nourished and relaxed. Making the effort to create precious moments of closeness and intimacy, which the two of you alone can enjoy, will keep the sparkle in your relationship.*

Sex in Maturity

Sexuality is not the sole prerogative of the young and there is no reason why people in their mature years should not continue to enjoy a happy sex life. Indeed, there are aspects of ageing that may actually enhance a sexual relationship, and research shows that even very elderly people can retain a healthy libido. While certain changes do occur in the sexual responses and reproductive organs of men and women as they grow older, if people can accept and adapt to them both physically and psychologically, then age itself does not preclude the capacity to be sexually fulfilled.

If a woman is past the menopause and no longer concerned about issues of pregnancy or contraception, she may feel more free to enjoy sex. Studies show that many women actually become more orgasmic in the later years of their lives, compared to when they were younger. However, as a man gets older he will often need more time and extra stimulation before he is able to get an erection.

If his partner is able to respond positively to this natural process of change, she may enjoy taking a more active and creative role than ever before in initiating the love play between them.

As people age, particularly if couples have been in a relationship for many years, their sexuality often becomes less focused on the act of penetration alone and more open to other forms of sensual and tactile contact, such as hugging, kissing, and loving caresses.

Even if a couple no longer desire penetrative intercourse, or if it is no longer possible because of health reasons, they can still pleasure each other with alternative forms of erotic love, such as oral sex and masturbation. In ways such as these, the physical intimacy between partners can actually develop as they grow older together and embrace a whole new sensuality that may have been missing in their earlier days.

Overcoming Taboos

One of the main problems facing the older generation is society's attitude towards sex and ageing. It is as if sex is seen as the domain of the young and beautiful alone, and that there is something indecent or embarrassing in acknowledging that older people may also have sexual needs.

Age and Intimacy
The twilight years of a relationship may allow a couple to discover a new level of intimacy.

Many older people feel embarrassed about revealing their sexual needs, finding it easier to repress them, and resign themselves to the commonly held opinion that at their age they should be "beyond it". Unfortunately, this view may prevent a mature couple seeking the specialist help they may need to resolve their physical and psychological sexual concerns. Even in long-term relationships, partners may give up all forms of physical intimacy because they feel unable to surmount these problems.

Many members of the older generation may believe that certain practices, such as oral sex and masturbation, are harmful, disgusting or even perverted. It is unlikely that, at this point in their lives, their views are going to change. However, oral sex is an excellent addition to a couple's love life, when sexual functioning is otherwise impaired by the ageing process or arousal responses have begun to slow down. An older man may find that he is more easily aroused and can maintain his erection better if his partner is willing to perform fellatio on him or to apply manual stimulation, strokes and caresses to his penis and testicles.

In a woman's case, after the menopause, her vagina may undergo various physical changes, losing much of its lubrication and elasticity. This can cause her discomfort in penetrative intercourse and reduce her enjoyment of sex. These changes are not related to her libido, which can still function healthily, and ageing should not affect the responsiveness of her clitoris, which is her most erotically sensitive organ. Cunnilingus is an excellent option in lovemaking, and one way that her partner can continue to give her sexual satisfaction.

Prostate Problems

Many men, particularly in their later years, experience urinary problems due to the enlargement of the prostate gland, which can obstruct the flow of urine. This can be rectified by medication, surgery, or by other forms of therapy. Men are often reluctant to seek treatment when they first realize they are having difficulty urinating, usually out of embarrassment. However, it is important to seek medical advice at the earliest opportunity, because delay risks serious complications, such as bladder infections and kidney damage. Treatment should not necessarily affect a man's sexual functioning, although a possible side-effect of prostate surgery is retrograde ejaculation, in which semen is propelled backwards into the bladder, rather than being expelled from the body.

The risk of cancer of the prostate also increases with age. This is one of the most common forms of cancer found in men but it responds well to treatment if detected in the early stages. Symptoms, if any, may be the same as for an enlarged prostate, and so this is another reason why it is important to seek medical advice if you experience problems urinating. Treatment carries some risk of infertility and impotence.

Changing Sexual Health

Health issues are the most significant factor in causing diminished sexual response as we grow older. It is natural for some people, as they age, to become less interested in sex. However, a sudden loss of libido, in men or women, could be due to illness or other physiological factors, and this should always be checked out with a doctor. Certain medications can inhibit sexual response, as can medical conditions such as diabetes, cardio-vascular diseases, and prostate disorders. Some women experience a loss of sexual feeling after the menopause, but this is by no means inevitable, and many women actually feel more sexual at this time than they did before.

However, there are natural changes in sexual response and functioning which occur as part of the ageing process. In themselves these do not necessarily prevent men or women from continuing to enjoy a happy sex life, especially if they are able to adapt to these changes and have an understanding partner who is also willing to explore new ways of enhancing the sexual relationship.

A man's reproductive capacity can remain throughout his life, although a decline in testosterone levels in later years may decrease his sperm production. However, as some famous men, such as Clint Eastwood or Anthony Quinn, have demonstrated in recent years, age is no bar to becoming a father. As he gets older, a man may find that he is slower to become aroused, and that his erection is less firm. He may take longer to ejaculate when making love, and may ejaculate with less frequency than when he was younger. Also, the refractory, or recovery, phase between each ejaculation will increase, and it may take several hours or even days before he can be aroused again.

There may also be psychological reasons for a man's changing sexual

Enjoying Leisure Together

▶ *Many couples, in their later years, have the opportunity to spend more leisure time together, free from work pressures or the demands of childrearing. This gives them more chance to enjoy each other's company so that their bond of affection and intimacy can deepen.*

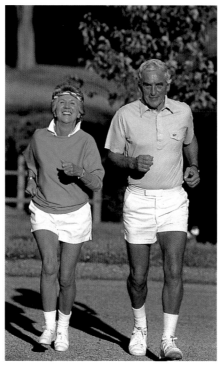

responses as he gets older. Many men equate their sense of virility and potency with their earning capacity and careers. When a man retires from work, he may feel that he is no longer useful and this can adversely affect his sexual performance. It is important for a man to maintain and develop absorbing or worthwhile interests and take up pursuits which will help him re-establish his self-esteem. Talking over these issues with an understanding partner, who can reassure him that he is still a real man in her regard, or discussing his problems with a counsellor, can help him to come to terms with his new role in life.

A woman will experience far more dramatic hormonal changes than a man as she ages. This change can herald a whole new phase in a woman's life, and can instil in her a range of emotions. She may feel that she is finally her own woman; many women consider the post-menopausal years to be the best time of their lives. This may also be tinged with a sense of loss that a certain aspect of her feminine role has gone for ever.

On average, the onset of the menopause occurs at around the age of 50 (although it can begin much earlier or later) and takes around two to five years to complete. During this time, there will be dramatic hormonal fluctuations

in the woman's body, and her oestrogen levels will steadily decline. Menstruation often becomes irregular, and there may be times when her periods are close together with a heavier than usual menstrual flow, and then more widely spaced, with only a very light showing of blood. Excessive bleeding or other menstrual problems should be investigated by a doctor to rule out possible disorders.

The menopause can affect women very differently, partly due to psychological factors such as whether they are mentally well prepared for the change, their attitude towards growing older and no longer being fertile, and the symptoms experienced during this process. Some women travel through this time without a backward glance, and suffer few of the more uncomfortable side-effects.

Many women, however, experience one or more unpleasant physical and psychological symptoms which can be directly related to the hormonal changes. These can include

hot flushes and night sweats, palpitations and anxiety attacks, loss of concentration, mood swings, lethargy, vaginal dryness and thinning of the vaginal tissues. In some women, the reduced oestrogen levels leads to osteoporosis, a thinning of the bones caused by calcium loss, leading to increased risk of fractures.

However, it is important that women realize the menopause in itself is not an illness but a natural part of the female life process. At the same time, no woman should hesitate in seeking medical advice if she is suffering from any of the debilitating symptoms described above.

Many doctors recommend that women take hormone replacement therapy (HRT) to safeguard their health during the menopause and even for a longer duration, while other medical experts disagree. The pros and cons of HRT are still being debated in the medical world. HRT will usually alleviate the physical side-effects of menopause, and is effective in reducing the risk of developing osteoporosis and heart disease.

Whether or not a woman chooses to take HRT, she should ensure that her lifestyle is balanced and healthy. A good nutritious diet, plenty of exercise, avoiding smoking and keeping alcohol intake to sensible levels will all enhance her state of well-being at this special time in her life.

As a woman ages, she may notice some change in her sexual organs and sexual responses. As oestrogen levels drop, it is possible that her vaginal secretions will decrease, and the vaginal lining will become thinner and so more vulnerable to tears and infection. To reduce friction and soreness during intercourse, she can use a lubricating jelly or obtain a locally applied oestrogen cream. She may also notice that, as she ages, her arousal responses are less intense, not because of a lack of desire, but because of physiological changes. There is no reason for her to become less orgasmic, although her climaxes may not seem as powerful as when she was younger.

For various medical reasons, a doctor may recommend that a woman undergoes a hysterectomy but it is advisable to seek a second medical opinion regarding the suitability of this operation in her circumstances. While a hysterectomy is more common once women have reached their forties and beyond, it may sometimes be necessary to carry out this procedure in a younger woman.

Once a woman has had a hysterectomy she is no longer able to have children, and if both ovaries are removed, she will become menopausal. In these circumstances, hormone replacement therapy is usually offered to the woman by her doctor. While a hysterectomy is a major surgical procedure, a healthy woman should recover well within six weeks of the operation if she is able to receive the adequate after-care and rest she needs.

A hysterectomy does not have to mean the end of a woman's sex life or capacity to enjoy sexual or orgasmic pleasure, although in some cases, women do report that the intensity of their orgasmic contractions reduces slightly. If a woman has to undergo a hysterectomy, it is important that she realizes the operation does not make her less feminine in any way.

Life Without Sex

For some people, sexual passion declines quite naturally after a certain age, and not only are they happy to accept this, they may even find it a relief. The freedom from being driven by sexual desires which had to be fulfilled can open up a whole new vista on life, allowing that person time to relax into other pleasures and pursuits. If this happens mutually within a partnership, the couple may find that their relationship changes to allow greater compatibility and growth in other areas of their lives.

If one partner loses the sex drive, while the other retains an active libido, they obviously need to talk about their incompatible desires and try to find a compromise. A couple who face this dilemma may also benefit from counselling to help them confront the changing nature of their relationship and enable them to acknowledge their own and each other's needs.

Sometimes the end of penetrative sex in a relationship can open up new horizons of loving sensual contact and deepening companionship through which both people can derive even greater emotional nourishment than before. For some people, to whom sex was more of a chore than a pleasure, the cessation of their sex lives can feel liberating.

There are circumstances, of course, when the loss of a sex life in the later years of life is not a matter of choice. Death, divorce, or separation may leave one partner alone, and often as we grow older, it becomes less possible or desirable to form new partnerships. Many people, from middle age to elderly years, face the prospect of spending the rest of their lives without a sexual companion. In a situation like this it is important to assess one's real needs and hopes, rather than abandon the idea of finding a new partner.

Some people take active measures, joining dating agencies or broadening their recreational activities to make new acquaintances, and achieve success in doing so. Others learn to accept their single status. Even so, it is still possible to keep the flame of sexual energy burning bright.

Dancing, having fun, sharing good times with friends, receiving a massage, cuddles and hugs from people who care, all help to keep sensual and sexual vitality alive. Masturbation is also a way to achieve release from sexual tension, but it can also be much more than that. Self-pleasuring can be a way of nurturing oneself, if time is taken to touch the whole body with care and love and it is done without haste, guilt or judgement.

Getting older, with or without a partner, does not mean that you can no longer enjoy the sensual and sexual pleasures of your body if you so desire. It is good and healthy for you to acknowledge and enjoy your sexuality, whatever your age.

A New Beginning?

◀ *Being alone need not be the same as being lonely. It is never too late to form a new relationship, perhaps as fulfilling as any you've known before.*

Touch & Sensual Massage

Introducing sensual massage as a regular event in a relationship is one of the most effective ways of enhancing physical and emotional communication. The loving and confident stroking of hands upon the skin, the way they mould into the body's curves, and the gentle palpation of muscles and tissues speak volumes in the silent language of touch about your innermost feelings for each other.

A sensual massage can help you and your partner unwind from the stresses of the day, creating a precious opportunity to relax and enjoy each other's company. A massage can be offered as a spontaneous gesture to ease a partner's pain or tension. You may want to give a soothing face massage, to relieve stress, anxiety or headache, or focus your strokes on the back, shoulders, and neck, to alleviate muscular aches

Loving Therapy

 Massage is a loving and therapeutic process which relieves tension in body and mind, and so allows more freedom to enjoy spontaneous interaction. By taking turns to massage each other, both partners can learn to enjoy sharing the roles of giving and receiving pleasure.

and strains. You can pamper your partner by offering her a luxurious foot or hand massage.

The session may evolve into a truly sensuous affair, involving flowing caresses of the whole body from top to toe. A massage can include a variety of strokes, from soft, languid touches to firm, invigorating movements. The beauty of massage is that its motions are like notes of music or the steps of a dance, varied enough to enable you to always respond creatively to your partner's changing needs and moods.

It may become a prelude to a loving and sexual encounter so that the whole body is more ready and responsive to pleasure and erotic feelings. Sensual massage helps to build physical and emotional trust because one partner surrenders his or her

Emotional Nourishment

▶ *Massage is the perfect medium for close physical contact at times when the libido of one or both partners is low, or there is a sexual dysfunction or physical condition that is inhibiting or preventing full sexual intercourse. By remaining in touch with one another's bodies, the essential emotional nourishment which ensues from physical intimacy can continue, thus avoiding a build-up of frustration, need and feelings of isolation. The strokes can release muscular tension from those areas of the body closely associated with sexual response, helping your partner to feel more alive and receptive to her sexual feelings.*

body into the hands of the other, while the person giving the massage must learn to respect and tune in to its innate needs and responses.

Touch as a Healing Force

The most important healing element in any massage is the power of loving touch. Touch is known as the mother of the senses, being the first to develop in the human embryo and in all other species, and the one on which all the other senses are based. The tactile sense resides in the skin, that miraculous organ covering the entire body. By means of its countless nerve endings, which respond to a whole variety of pressures from pain to pleasure, the skin relays messages through the central nervous system to the brain, transmitting information about the external world beyond its frontiers. A loving touch which brings reassurance and joy to the skin will ultimately infuse the whole body with a feeling of well-being.

Touch is an essential form of nourishment for the psychosomatic processes of body, mind and spirit throughout our lives. Adequate loving touch, in the form of affectionate caressing, hugging, stroking, cuddling and kissing, is vital in the early stages of infancy for the healthy development of a growing child. Through these pleasurable skin sensations, the infant can begin to define its sense of self-worth, and to develop an understanding and an appreciation of its own body.

Touch deprivation in early childhood can retard physical and emotional growth, potentially leading to health, behavioural and sexual problems in later years. Lack of adequate touch, even in adulthood, can rob someone of the feelings of vitality and ease within the body. This will often manifest itself as an

Healing Touch

▲ By letting massage become a regular feature of a relationship, partners can learn to develop whole body sensuality, increase skin sensitivity to both external stimuli and internal feelings, and to develop a growing confidence and trust in the nurturing and healing qualities of touch.

inability to express or receive affection adequately.

Loving touch, through the medium of massage, will help to heal old emotional wounds whose memories remain locked within the body, establishing a new and positive sense of body image, confidence and responsiveness to physical sensuality.

When couples experiment with touch techniques they discover, often to their surprise, that to give a massage is as satisfying as receiving one. This is because by touching and using your feeling senses, you open up the depths of your own emotions, and have a means to express them. Within a massage sequence, you can be playful, tender, strong, creative and loving. By coming to know and understand another's body, you begin to become more aware of your own physical needs.

It is important, however, to give massage only when willing to do so, for it is a caring act and the message imparted from your hands always

Tender Outpouring

▲ By opening your heart and pouring tenderness into your hands as you stroke each part of his body, you can impart to him a deeply nurturing sense of love and care which will increase his feelings of physical well-being and of self-worth. Massage expresses and heightens emotional bonding in a unique way.

Fluid Movements

▲ In an intimate and sensual massage, use your hands, forearms, and other parts of your body to stroke the skin, letting the touches flow like water over the body. At some moments it will seem as if the two bodies have melted and merged into one another, dissolving the physical boundaries between you.

Overture to Lovemaking

▼ *If both of you are clear that a sensual massage is a luxurious prelude to lovemaking, then once you have warmed and relaxed the whole body, you can stroke over the erogenous areas to increase excitement.*

conveys your innermost feelings. Equally, it is important to know whether the massage you plan is purely for sensual pampering, relaxing or revitalizing, or whether it is an erotic encounter as a prelude to making love.

Naturally, if there is mutual consent, a massage may transform from one experience into the other, but it is wrong to use the situation as a means of seduction if your partner has not given you clear signals of consent. If the massage is intended purely to soothe, comfort and relax, or your partner is unwilling to engage in sexual activity, then it is better to avoid direct contact with the genitalia or other erogenous areas which could provoke an unwanted sexual response in either of you.

Selecting the Oils

Choose a light, preferably unrefined vegetable oil for lubrication, such as grapeseed, safflower or sunflower oil, to which you can add a much richer oil, such as almond, avocado or jojoba.

Learn about the soothing, romantic and erotic qualities of essential oils, so that you can create aromatic blends to enhance the sensuous mood of your massage. Place your oil in a ceramic bowl or a bottle that will allow you to pour the right amount into your hands. Warm the oil before applying it. Keep tissues or towels nearby for oil spillage or to wipe your hands.

If your partner does not like oil on his skin, then use a body lotion with nourishing skin properties. Talcum powder can also be used, though its dryness will prevent you from performing the flowing, soporific motions of a truly sensual massage.

Learning to receive massage is also a helpful process for those people who predominantly identify with the role of the main giver in a relationship, often unconsciously taking control of events and denying the other partner the chance to reciprocate love and concern. To receive massage is one of the few occasions in life where all you need to do is become totally receptive. Even in lovemaking, there is usually a constant interaction of activity.

To allow yourself to become passive, and simply receive touch,

means you must open yourself up to a certain degree of trust and vulnerability and this, in itself, is a gift which you can offer to your partner. Make sure you take it in turns to give and receive massage so that you can both learn from all aspects of the experience.

The Strokes of Massage

Confidence, quality of touch in your hands and sensitivity to your partner's body are essential if the massage is to be mutually satisfying and pleasurable. But do give each other scope to experiment with different strokes, pressures and touches. Treat the whole experience as a game, make it fun, and tell each other what feels good. Give one another a chance to explore the techniques without being too directive, but make your feelings clear to your partner if you do not feel comfortable with what is happening to your body.

There are some basic rules to follow and certain strokes to learn that will improve the experience and enhance your mutual repertoire of techniques. By learning how to apply different movements and pressures you will be able to give the right massage for the occasion. You can also expand on your techniques by reading suitable massage manuals, or participating in a massage workshop with your partner.

The first step is to lubricate the area of the body you are about to massage. Pour a little oil into one palm and then rub both hands together to warm it before spreading the lubricant with soft, free-flowing motions, using the flat surface of your palms.

Apply sufficient oil to ensure your hands slide sensuously over the skin. These soporific strokes will help your

Liquid Warmth

◀ *Your liquid movements as you spread the oil will warm the muscles, boost the circulation, and prepare the body's tissues for other strokes. There is no need to hurry this part of the massage as it will give you both time to relax, focus your attention, and tune in to one another.*

Following the Contours

▼ *Allow all the tension to leave your hands so that they are able to glide, melt and sculpt the underlying contours and curves of your partner's body and bring to both him and yourself a much clearer definition of its shape and structure.*

Close Contact

◀ *By straddling your partner, you can comfortably enfold the circumference of his back in one long flowing sweep, stroking your hands up along his spine, over his shoulders and back down the sides of his body. Your physical closeness will add to the sensuality of the massage, but take care to support your own weight.*

Rounded Movements

▶ *Sensual massage movements should be smooth and rounded and never finish abruptly mid-way on the body. Always glide your hands around the body's contours, such as the shoulders or hips, or sweep them out along the limbs.*

Circle Strokes

1 *To circle stroke, place both hands flat and parallel on the body, with fingers pointing away from you. Your hands should be about 10cm/4in apart. With a steady pressure, begin to slide both hands in a circular clockwise motion with your right hand leading the movement.*

Lift and Pass

2 *Lift your right hand slightly away from the body, crossing it over the top of your left hand which continues to circle underneath.*

Completing the Circle

3 *As your left hand completes its circle, your right hand drops down to perform a half-circle, then lifts off again to let your left hand pass. Now repeat this sequence.*

partner forget any stressful thoughts he might have and become more receptive to your touch.

You can create a truly relaxing and sensual massage using only soft gliding strokes in a variety of unbroken and flowing motions that embrace the whole body. By letting your hands slide from the back to the legs in simple easy stretches, or, when stroking the front of the body, from the thighs to the belly, you will bring a sense of unity and integration to your partner's body.

Circle and Fan Strokes

Circle and fan strokes stretch and ease the tension out of the body's soft tissues, bringing a lovely fluid and hypnotic movement to a session of sensual massage.

Circle strokes are applied to any broad surface area of the body, such as the back and sides of the body, the thighs, belly and chest. The art of this stroke is to keep it constantly spiralling over the skin until you are ready to move with an unbroken motion into the next sequence of strokes. The circle stroke is shown (*left*) in three stages.

Fanning Strokes

◄ *Fanning motions can be applied upwards or downwards. Once your hands have reached the base of the back on a downwards sequence, return to the top of the spine by gliding them up along the sides of the ribcage.*

Fan Strokes

1 *To fan upwards, place both hands flat, pointing to the head, on each side of the lower end of the spine.*

Fanning Out

2 *Glide both your hands upwards for a distance of about 15cm/6in before fanning them out towards the sides of the body.*

Gliding Downwards

3 *Mould both hands firmly to the sides of the body and pull downwards. Then, with a turn of the wrists, glide your hands towards the centre of the back before stroking upwards again.*

Essential Oils

All that is necessary for sensual massage is a basic carrier oil, such as sunflower or almond oil. But by blending in a few drops of one or more essential oils you can make the massage a truly memorable experience. Essential oils have their own unique therapeutic qualities – some are highly beneficial in relieving stress, for example. You and your partner should both decide on the blend of essential oils, otherwise if one of you finds an aroma unpleasant the massage will not be so pleasurable. Some oils such as rose, jasmine, sandalwood, rosewood, and the exotic ylang ylang enjoy a widespread appeal.

Warning: Essential oils are highly concentrated and should never be spread directly onto the skin. Always blend them with a suitable carrier oil first. For a whole body massage, add 10-15 drops of one, two or three essential oils to five teaspoons of base carrier oil.

Fan strokes are applied to most areas of the body with an upward, flowing and steady pressure using the surface of both palms. One fan stroke should merge into the next in a constant upward movement, which boosts the circulation towards the heart. When your hands reach to the top of a body part, fan them out to the sides and slide them back down to repeat the sequence. The fan stroke over the lower back is shown opposite in three stages.

Invigorating Strokes

Invigorating strokes add variety and spice to your sensual massage. They have a revitalizing effect on the system, boosting the blood circulation, loosening stiff muscles and ridding the tissues of trapped toxins. Your partner will enjoy the stimulat-

Soothing Strokes

◄ *Large circle strokes on the abdomen are very soothing, helping your partner breathe more deeply, so that she is more in touch with her sexual and emotional feelings. Always approach the abdomen sensitively as it is a vulnerable area.*

ing effect and the sensation of different pressures. Introduce friction, kneading and percussion strokes to the massage, once the muscles are warm and relaxed.

Always precede and follow invigorating movements with sensual strokes to soothe the skin and to integrate the part of the body under focus with the surrounding area. Friction grinds the tissue towards the bone and is excellent for relieving specific areas of tension. Pressure is applied slowly and sensitively from the heels of the hand, the thumbs, fingertips, or knuckles. The movement can be a steady slide, a short stretch, or small circular motions in which the pressure is greater on the outward half of the circle. Use friction whenever you are working close to the bone, such as alongside the

Spinal Relaxation

◄ *The spine is often one of the most tense areas of the body. The deeper stretching movement of a friction stroke over the muscles and ligaments running alongside the vertebrae will help to relieve stiffness from your partner's back, enabling him to relax more fully and enjoy the massage. In this movement, the thumb pads are pressed slowly at the top of the back into the grooves either side of the spine, while the hands rest on the body. Lean your weight steadily into the stroke as you slide your thumbs down towards the base of the back. Then glide your hands around his hips, up the sides of the ribcage and over the shoulders to repeat the whole sequence with a deeper level of pressure. To vary the stroke, make small circular movements with your thumbs moving down each side of the spine.*

Fleshy Zones

◄ *Kneading strokes are perfect for the fleshy erogenous zones of the buttocks and thighs, as the invigorating action helps to release tension from their large muscles and stimulate the sensory nerves that affect sexual response. When massaging the buttocks, begin with smooth, gliding motions that shape their ample contours, and then proceed with the kneading.*

Brisk Strokes

▼ *The brisk staccato movements of hacking can be a fun addition to sensual massage, particularly over the buttocks and thighs, as they will enliven the skin and may even stimulate your partner erotically. However, if he is feeling particularly vulnerable, or the mood of the massage is very relaxed, save these strokes for times when invigorating stimulation is the desired result.*

spine, around the shoulder blades, under or over the scalp, or on the hands, feet and face.

Kneading is applied to the fleshy parts of the body such as the shoulders, sides of the body, buttocks and thighs. Kneading, as the name suggests, replicates the action of a baker kneading dough, and is performed by scooping up and squeezing a portion of flesh between the fingers, heel and thumb of one hand before pushing it towards the other hand. The waiting hand then repeats the action, and in this way the flesh is rolled back and forth between both hands. Work thoroughly over an area, ensuring that your wrists and shoulders remain relaxed so that the kneading has a fluid and wave-like motion.

Percussion strokes are rapid, vibratory movements used to revitalize the system and tone up the skin by enriching the blood supply to its nerve endings. There are a variety of percussion strokes, all made with one hand following the other in quick succession to strike the flesh briskly before flicking immediately back off the skin. They feel best when applied to fleshy areas and should never be used directly over the bones.

Pummelling is done by rhythmically striking the sides of loosely made fists against the body, while hacking is performed with a series of gentle chopping movements made from the sides of open, straight hands. Relax your wrists so the percussion strokes remain bouncy but not heavy-handed.

Maintain Good Posture

Whether you are kneeling, sitting or standing while massaging your partner, it is always important to take care of your own posture, pausing to relax and breathe deeply whenever you feel tense. By remaining at ease in your body and breathing, your own vitality is sustained throughout the massage. This boosts your enjoyment of giving the massage and brings a comforting warmth and vitality to your hands. As a consequence, good posture improves the quality of your massage strokes.

Preparation for Massage

When you set the scene for a luxurious and sensual massage, take time to create a romantic ambience so that your partner will know this is a special occasion. Place flowers around the room for their delicate aroma and colourful effects, and light candles to create a mellow mood, putting them at a safe distance from the place you are giving the massage.

You should cover the mattress or surface you are working on with fresh, clean sheets, and also keep extra sheets and towels close by in case your partner gets cold. Have your favourite romantic style of music playing softly in the background but take care not to let the sounds invade the natural rhythm of your massage strokes.

Choose the setting for massage carefully, so both of you can relax fully. The room must be warm and draught-free if clothes are to be removed. Try to ensure privacy so the person receiving the massage has a chance to put all concerns aside, and the one giving it can devote his or her attention to the session.

In a full-body massage, both partners need a firm base such as a futon, a layer of foam, or a strong mattress to support their body weight under the pressure of strokes and movements. Folded blankets, a covered sleeping bag or firm cushions laid on the floor will also suffice. Towels and oils should be kept close at hand.

Spontaneous Massage

Different locations and occasions can turn a massage into a spontaneous treat. For instance, when bathing together you have the perfect opportunity for an impromptu massage, especially as your skin-to-skin

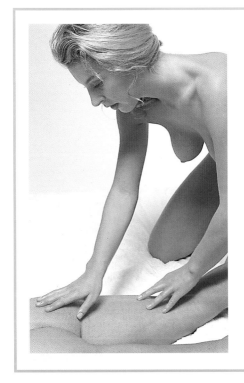

The Gossamer Touch

Feather touches are a sensual, skin-teasing way to carry out a series of strokes over any area. Using only the minimum of pressure from your fingertips, stroke very lightly over the skin, one hand following the other, and moving in one direction at a time. This will activate the skin's peripheral nerve endings, exquisitely heightening its sensitivity. Some people may find the touch just too light and ticklish, while others love its euphoric effects and would quite happily surrender to a whole body massage of these strokes alone.

Massage Table

◀ *You can use a table for a massage base if it is sufficiently long and strong to take the size and weight of your partner, and narrow enough for you to reach her body. Pad it with blankets or cushions for comfort. A table of the right height and dimensions has the advantage of allowing you more freedom of movement, although it will inhibit close physical contact.*

contact will feel deliciously natural and uninhibited. In the bath, take turns to give each other a shoulder and neck massage. Your soothing strokes will assist the therapeutic qualities of warm water as it draws the tension out of the muscles.

If you have a fireplace, take the opportunity to massage your partner in front of a lighted hearth at the end of the evening or after a bath. The heat of a fire adds a primal earthiness to your nakedness and physical contact, and you can give a full body sensual massage to your partner as he or she lies on folded blankets or a thin mattress in front of the flickering flames. Or simply take it in turns to give a head, neck and shoulder massage to relax your partner before going to sleep.

Lather as Lubricant
 In the bath, the rich soapy lather on her skin acts as a lubricant for you to glide your hands soothingly over the top of her back and shoulders. Then relax her spine with friction strokes. Hook your fingers over her shoulders and work your thumbs in small circular motions up alongside the bones.

Friction Rub
▶ *Use a loofah or soap glove to massage the skin. The gentle friction leaves it soft and glowing. Rub over the chest and arms, and then the back and shoulders.*

Relaxing Aromas
▲ *You can add a few drops of essential oils into your basic oil to increase the relaxing effect of this fireside massage. Use soft, sensual strokes to sculpt the upper back and ease the tension from the shoulders and neck.*

Targeting Tensions
▲ *Focus on tight areas between the shoulder blades, and at the base of the neck. Hook your fingers over his shoulders, and sink your thumb pads into the muscles, then use small circular motions over each tense spot in turn.*

Tingling Vibrations
▲ *Hack briskly and firmly over the top of the shoulders and down along the sides of the shoulder blades, but avoid striking the spine. The rapid vibrations will loosen stiff shoulders and leave the skin flushed and tingling.*

Soothing the Mind
▲ *A head massage can calm the mind when your partner is feeling under stress. Firmly circle the fingertips of both hands over his entire scalp, then comb your fingers through his hair to complete your fireside massage.*

Tender Loving Care

Some people find it difficult to express their love verbally. Often, a tender touch conveys these feelings more directly than words. It is an instinctive human response to embrace a person as a gesture of affection, to take hold of the hand to comfort, or to soothe away pain with a gentle rub. When you make love, the way you touch the whole body is as important as the sexual act itself, because it communicates your loving feelings.

A sensual massage is a wonderful opportunity to give and receive tender, loving care but even if you do not have time for a full-body session, you can still pamper your partner with shorter programmes of massage which will leave him or her feeling cherished and relaxed. At the end of a tiring day, a twenty-minute massage is still an excellent treat.

A foot massage will dissolve stress and soothe body and mind. The soft strokes over the feet have a calming effect, while the stronger pressures will boost low energy levels. Massage one foot at a time, and spread a little lotion over the top and sole with gliding, sensual strokes. When the foot is warm and supple, stroke your fingertips or thumb pads around the sides, front and back of the ankle to release any tension. Press or slide your thumbs firmly all over the sole to stimulate its countless nerve endings.

Pay attention to the toes as touch here is surprisingly sensual. Palpate each toe gently between thumb and finger, then slide your little finger between each toe and rub the soft webs of skin with little corkscrew motions. Add the strokes shown here to your massage and then repeat them all on the other foot.

Cradling the Foot

▶ *When you have completed the strokes on one foot, cradle it between your hands for a while, focusing all your attention towards your touch. The soft, enfolding embrace of the foot will deeply relax your partner.*

Position for Foot Massage

◀ *Foot massage gives you a chance to relax together, to chat and catch up on the news of the day while enjoying physical contact at the same time. Make sure your partner is sitting comfortably while she receives the massage, and her leg is supported by cushions. Position yourself so you can easily apply strokes to both sides of her foot.*

Tension-free Toes

▲ *The toes tend to retain tension, which adds stress to the posture. Stretching them brings relief to the whole body. After pressing gently over the toe, hold it between your thumb and index finger, and pull steadily along its length from the base to its tip. You will need to swap the position of your hands to stretch the big toe.*

Feather Touches

◀ *Feather-stroke down the leg and over the foot several times towards the end of the massage if your partner enjoys these exhilarating, skin-tingling touches.*

Many of the strokes used on the feet can be adapted to a hand massage. If your partner's work is manual, or involves gripping a pen or using a keyboard all day, a hand massage can alleviate the strain of repetitive movements which accumulates in the tendons and muscles. Make sure he is sitting or lying comfortably, so that his shoulders and arms are relaxed while you massage his hands.

A face massage is one of the most intimate and loving ways to give pleasure through touch. Use soft caresses to calm and reassure, and steady, firm pressures to relieve

Loving Lotion
▲ Hand-to-hand contact conveys a silent message of love, friendship and support. Spread lotion over the hand with gliding strokes and then hold it between the warmth of your palms.

Slide and Stretch
◄ Make short, firm, sliding strokes with one thumb following the other, over the palm and up to the wrist to stretch away tension. Rest the back of the hand against your fingers. Rest his arm on a cushion during the massage.

tension spots in this most revealed and revealing part of the body.

Every thought and emotion expresses itself in the face and, often, its muscles tighten to present an acceptable mask to the world. When your lover comes home, help him to become more vulnerable and allow his true feelings to rise to the surface by stroking away the stress.

To give a face massage, kneel or sit behind your partner's head so that it rests between your legs. Place a cushion under his head to take the

strain off the back of his neck. Begin by cupping your hands very lightly over each side of his jaw and letting them rest there in a calm and still hold for up to a count of ten. Then stroke with the palms of both hands continuously, one after the other, along the jawbone from the chin to the ear until you feel the whole area relaxing under these loving caresses.

Take the lobes of the ears between thumbs and fingertips and gently press them, then make tiny circle

strokes all along the rims of the ears. Sweep your fingers in outward-flowing circles over both cheeks to move and loosen tense muscles. Follow this by tracing the fingertips of one hand lightly round and round the sensuous curves of the lips.

Using the tips of the first two fingers of each hand, stroke deftly around the eye socket up to ten times from the outer bridge of the nose to the edge of the temples, continuing lightly over the top of the cheekbones back towards the sides of the nose.

Steady Pressure

◀ *When massaging the face, your strokes should be smooth, steady and consistent. Apply a gentle but firm pressure as you move over tension areas, such as directly under the cheekbones. In this movement, your hands softly clasp the sides of his face while your thumbs slide down the edges of the nose and continue stretching outwards under the bone. Lighten the pressure as you get closer to the ears. Draw your hands lightly over the head before repeating the stroke twice more.*

Help for Headaches

◀ *To relieve a tension headache, place your thumbs over the centre of the forehead just above the eyebrows while resting your hands on the sides of the face. Steadily draw your thumbs outwards over the brow, completing the stroke with a sweep of the temples. Continue repeating this stroke to cover the whole forehead, moving up a little at a time until you reach the hair line.*

Glide your fingertips smoothly in clockwise motions around the temples, increasing the pressure slightly on the outward sweep. Now soothe the brow by softly drawing each hand consecutively across the forehead from the opposite-side temple, repeating these hypnotic movements for up to two minutes. Then work the fingertips of both hands simultaneously in small circles over the scalp as if shampooing the hair.

Complete the face massage with a still and tender hold by placing your thumbs over the centre of his crown, so that his head nestles between your hands and your fingers lay symmetrically over his temples. Close your eyes and focus your attention on your hands to pour your loving feelings into them. After a minute or two, slowly withdraw your hands from the head but sit quietly with your partner so you can both enjoy these precious and peaceful moments together.

Soothing Strokes

◀ *Your partner will love the feeling as your fingers comb through his hair, as if they are drawing the last of the day's stresses out of his mind and body. It is a very soothing motion to add to the last few strokes of a face and head massage.*

Games & Exercises

Games and exercises offer a great opportunity for you and your partner to relax and have fun together, while renewing your physical vitality as you breathe more deeply, tone up your muscles and stretch your joints. It is a chance to enjoy your own and your lover's body outside of sexual contact.

These exercises provide a non-threatening and playful opportunity in which to discover whether there are any subtle physical and psychological tensions within yourself and your relationship that may be inhibiting harmonious and spontaneous interaction. Tension often reflects an internal state of mind, such as a fear of letting go or of losing control, which shows itself outwardly as hesitation, resistance or even aggression.

The games will help you find a point of balance in yourself where you are at ease and relaxed within your body and mind. From this position you then co-operate with your partner, to find a mutual point of harmony and balance between you.

Before attempting the exercises, warm up with one or both of the two

Exercise One

1 Get the passive partner to stand in a balanced posture, feet a shoulder-width apart and knees flexed, taking a few moments to relax all joints. He then drops his head forwards and leans his upper body towards the ground. The head and neck hang relaxed between the shoulders, and his arms dangle loosely down. As the active partner, pummel briskly, one hand following the other, up along each side of his spine, and between the shoulder blades. Take care not to strike the spine itself.

Soothe the Spine

2 After the invigorating pummelling, soothe your partner's spine and back with overlapping strokes from the fingers of each hand. Start the motion from the lower back, drawing one hand after the other up along the spine and over the neck. Repeat this action several times.

Stimulating Strokes

3 Move to your partner's side and hack briskly over the large muscles of the buttocks to invigorate and stimulate this area and to loosen its tension. Aim for the fleshy areas, taking care not to strike the lower spine or pelvic bones. You can continue this hacking motion down to the thighs.

Friction Rub

4 Position yourself behind his posterior, and apply a friction rub over the kidney area to warm and revitalize the whole body. Using the flat surface of each hand alternately, briskly rub them back and forth for about thirty seconds to generate a tingling heat. Then, soothe the back with some sensual strokes. Now ask your passive partner to extend his upper body, uncoiling the spine slowly from its base, vertebra by vertebra. The last area to lift is the neck and head which then rests, relaxed and balanced, over the spine. Give him a few moments to experience this sensation of easy graceful length through the upper body.

Clear the Chest

5 Now ask your partner to expand his chest, by pushing his fists into his lower back, while letting his shoulders and head drop backwards. Encourage him to clear tension from his throat by emitting sounds while you pummel thoroughly over the chest. The pummelling dispels carbon dioxide from the lungs, helping him to breathe more deeply and to release sensations of tightness in the ribcage. When you have completed these strokes, your partner should stand straight and shake his arms and hands, and then legs and feet, to loosen up their joints.

Exercise Two

1 In the second warm-up exercise, the partner who is lying down first relaxes her whole body, and then focuses her breath and attention softly towards her abdomen. Lay your hands gently but with total presence on her belly to develop warmth and contact. Encourage her to become aware of her belly's expansion towards your hands with each inhalation, and its contraction with each exhalation.

Take the Weight

2 Cradle your partner's pelvis and lower abdomen between the reassuring contact of your hands, by slipping one hand beneath the lower back, and the other just above the pubic bone. Wait patiently for her to drop the weight of her back and pelvis into the support of your lower hand, while she directs her breathing and mental concentration to her pelvic girdle and genitals, allowing those areas to relax more with each cycle of breath.

Breathing Away Tension

3 Stress causes the diaphragm, the sheath of muscle separating the chest and the abdominal cavity, to tighten, constricting breathing, increasing feelings of anxiety and cutting you off from basic emotions. Scoop the hand which is closest to your partner's head under her body to rest beneath the middle of her back. Encourage her to consciously release the tension in her back towards this hand. Place the other hand softly over the diaphragm area, above the solar plexus, and just below the ribcage. Ask your partner to breathe gently into the area between your hands and allow her tension to melt with each exhalation.

ten-minute tactile contact programmes shown here. The first exercise uses some of the percussion strokes explained in Sensual Massage to enliven the body and help ease strain from the back, shoulders and chest. The second exercise encourages greater relaxation and more fullness of breath, while helping you to make a deeper connection with the abdominal and pelvic area, the centre of gravity and balance in your body.

Physical relaxation and emotional trust come from a sense of being at ease with your body and feelings, so you can trust your basic instincts. Those feelings are deeply rooted in the body, and in particular, within the abdominal region.

After each exercise, take some time to assimilate its effects, and discuss with each other what feelings or sensations occurred. Then you can reverse roles.

Developing Trust and Synchronicity

Fundamentally, the following exercises centre on developing trust and attaining synchronicity. Both factors represent a huge dynamic in any relationship. Our basis of trust develops within us as children through the experiences of our primary relationships, and is generally replayed unconsciously in other relationships throughout our adult lives. Learning to trust more does not mean that we must throw caution to the wind; our inner self-protection mechanisms have developed for good reason and need to be respected.

Through physical game-playing we can become aware of our fears about developing real trust – and the body is the most manifest place for this observation – and can sometimes gain insights into our earlier childhood experiences. We can then begin

Game One: Synchronizing

1 Both of you should squat, facing each other and maintaining eye contact, but with sufficient distance to let your arms stretch out to make contact. Keep your backs straight, and your neck and head loose and relaxed. Focus your breath and attention on your pelvic region to allow this point of gravity to give you balance. Let the genital area, and especially the anus, relax, and drop the weight of your buttocks towards the floor. Weight should be distributed evenly throughout the feet. Once you feel comfortable in your own squatting position, reach out and clasp each other's hands or wrists.

to undo some of our fears and inhibitions, while regaining more natural spontaneity. Awareness occurs the moment we draw something from the unconscious into our conscious minds, and is always the first point of any change.

By playing these games, you also learn how to become attentive and aware of whatever is happening, both within yourself and your partner. You cannot expect your lover to relax deeply and trust in the situation if you are self-absorbed, or your attention is wandering, or if you are neither sensitive nor receptive to the mental and bodily signals he or she is giving out.

Try not to overpower your partner, or demand results, and be patient whenever you meet a moment of physical or emotional resistance. Explore those experiences together, trying to gain insight into their

messages and learn from them. These games are intended to be fun and should not become a serious encounter, even if they evoke some profound feelings. They are an experiment, allowing you both to interchange constantly between passive and active roles, and to become confident and attuned to your bodies, so that you can develop a more harmonious relationship.

A successful relationship between two people also results when synchronicity is attained on energetic, physical and mental levels. Many couples are drawn to each other in the first place because of a certain rapport, although initially this may be an unconscious factor in their mutual attraction. There is a kind of ebb and flow in a happy relationship, where a balance exists between knowing when to take the lead and when to yield.

Push and Pull

2 When you are ready, begin to lever yourselves upwards from the squatting position. The thrust of the upwards movement should come from your leg muscles and hips, so always keep your spine lengthened and your shoulders relaxed. The art of this exercise is to find a mutual point of balance between you as you gently push and pull on each other to rise upwards. Too much or too little assertion from either partner will tip this delicate balance, causing one or both of you to topple over.

Lift and Descend

3 Raise up your bodies until you are both standing, then begin the process again as you lower yourselves back down to a squatting position. Repeat the exercise several times until you have found a fluid balance of movement between you.

Synchronicity is the moment when these two facets of the one phenomenon come together and form a unity of thought and action. Perhaps this can best be witnessed when two people dance together and their bodies flow as one motion, because they are able to respond equally to one another's subliminal signals indicating when to take the initiative and when to surrender to the movement.

This fine tuning manifests itself in bed too, when lovemaking can become a congruent interplay of

Game Two: Letting Go

1 In this exercise, your partner lies on the floor with her back relaxed and her legs raised in the air. Gently, but firmly, push both legs to one side of her body and then remove your hands.

Back Swing

2 When you have released contact, she then swings her legs back to a central position. At this point, decide on the direction of the next push so that one movement flows into another.

mind, heart and body, or adversely, a battleground of subtle domination, control, resistance or submission.

Synchronicity, which tends to exist naturally in the first stages of a relationship, should not be taken for granted. It can be lost as the individual personalities and egos emerge, or when either one or both partners becomes enmeshed in the normal stresses and strains of daily life.

The four exercises in this section will help you become more attuned to each other, as they require both trust and synchronicity while finding a harmonious balance between taking passive and active roles.

The first exercise involves squatting, the importance of which, as a pelvic floor exercise, has been fully explained in the section on

Change Directions

3 Try to use a whole range of directions, this time pushing the legs to the left side of the body. The side-to-side and back-and-forth movements of the legs will exercise and strengthen the abdominal muscles. Gently make her aware of whether she is resisting or aiding you as she should be yielding to these passive movements.

Exercises for Sexual Fitness. Turn it into a game with your partner, so that both of you can benefit from its muscle-strengthening and balancing effects, while making it a playful exercise of mutual movement coordination.

The next two games use a push-and-let-go technique, which requires the active person to take charge of moving the other's body, while the passive partner yields to the movement. The motions must be confident but gentle so your partner can trust you and relax. You must become sensitive to his or her body and its range of movement. If you are jerky, too fast, or too aggressive, your partner will resist you and tighten up. In the first exercise you work just with the legs, and in the second exercise you move the whole body.

The last exercise is a trust game in which you stand as a support for your partner as he or she falls backwards into your arms.

Reverse Roles

4 When you have completed a whole range of movements, swap roles. By pushing the legs towards the body you are giving a stretch to the lower back and hip joints.

Game Three: Taking Charge

1 This exercise is performed in a standing position. Ask your partner to stand in a relaxed posture so that she feels secure and balanced. She should close her eyes and focus on her breath and the sensations of movement. Position yourself behind her body and, with the lightest of touches, begin to direct her, pushing her gently to the side with one hand, and catching her with the other. Stay relaxed as you confidently take charge of her movements, keeping perfectly in tune with her sense of balance.

Gentle Rolling

2 Gracefully and quietly move around her body so that she is unable to guess the angle of the next movement. Roll her gently from side to side and back and forth, so that her body falls easily from one hand into the other.

Loosening Circles

3 Help her to loosen the hips and pelvis by circling this area between your hands. As she relaxes, and yields and allows her whole body to surrender to your hand directions, the movements can be gradually enlarged.

Learning to Surrender

▲ *Initially, your man may find it difficult to surrender his body to these movements, fearing he is too big or heavy to let you take charge. If he is able to relax and release body rigidity, you will be able to move him with ease.*

Game Four: Trust

1 This game is definitely about trust, and also requires the total attention of the active partner; only play it if you are confident about catching and supporting the weight of your partner's body. Ask her to stand in front of you, fully relaxed and with eyes closed. Position yourself behind, allowing enough space for her to fall back into your arms.

Falling for You

2 When she is ready, she allows herself to fall slowly backwards, trusting that you are there for her. The more physically relaxed she is able to remain, the easier it is for her to fall.

Safe Catch

3 As she tilts back, catch her securely in your arms, so that her upper back is supported and her head and neck rest against your chest or shoulder. Hold her against you for some moments, so she becomes aware of what she is feeling, then gently ease her back to a standing position. Repeat the exercise twice more.

Back To Back

Most of the time we relate to others face to face. We spend inordinate amounts of time taking care of the front, ensuring we present a good image to our partners or to the world at large. Normally, we have very little sense of ourselves as viewed from the backs of our bodies. It is to correct such a gap in our self-knowledge that this book has emphasized the great importance of touching, stroking and making sensual contact with the back of the body during foreplay and love-making, as well as dealing with the more obvious intimate and directly sexual areas located at the front.

The back acts as a protective shell, often harbouring tensions which shield a deeper level of vulnerability. If you have practised your sensual massage strokes on each other, you may have noticed how, once the muscles of the back are relaxed, the whole body seems to become more alive and sensitive. Often, touch, massage and contact to the back can help someone let go of their inner emotional tensions.

Here are some exercises you can enjoy with your partner to develop more familiarity with your own and each other's back. Through them, you develop a clearer feeling of its shape and structure and, therefore, a stronger sense of your body image.

In addition, these back-to-back exercises can help you dissolve the tensions which tend to keep you rigid, and allow you both to melt more with each other, both physically and emotionally.

Again, you need to be sensitive to each other and find a mutual point of balance, where your weight and movement are evenly and gently distributed. (It is not advisable to do these exercises if you are suffering from back problems of an acute or chronic nature.)

Begin by sitting with your backs to each other on a firm and supportive base, so that the surface of your backs and your spines are in comfortable contact. How much contact depends, of course, on the differences in your size and structure. It is important not to slump, but to keep your spines relaxed yet extended upwards.

Link your arms loosely together, and spend about three minutes directing your awareness and breath to areas of the back which feel tight and withholding, gradually allowing the tensions to melt.

Lean gently into each other, taking care not to burden your partner with your weight, especially if he or she is smaller or lighter than you. Close your eyes and begin to focus on the skin-to-skin contact of your backs, the shape and structure, how and where they fit together perfectly, and where there is tension. Imagine those tensions are beginning to dissolve so that both backs are merging together.

Start to sway gently together, finding a natural rhythm to your motion, and becoming more aware of the moments when the movements jar. Change the rhythm every so often, but always aim to remain harmoniously in tune with your partner's body.

Try to stay aware of any feelings which arise in you or you may be

Fitting Together
◄ *Bend your knees to lower your body so that she can fit her buttocks comfortably into the small of your back. Before moving, ensure that she is ready and relaxed for the lift.*

picking up from your partner as you let go of muscular tensions.

Now, sit silently together, eyes closed, but staying as deeply in tune with each other as possible for at least a minute. Once you are ready to separate, it is a good idea to discuss with each other what you experi-enced during this exercise, both in relation to your own body and your partner's body.

This back-to-back attunement game will prepare you for the spinal stretch exercise shown here, in which one partner lifts the other onto his or her back and balances the weight.

If you are lifting your partner, stabi-lize your own body by placing your feet a shoulder-width apart, and focus your breath towards your abdomen. This movement requires the recipient to trust the active partner enough to relax the weight of the whole back while being lifted upwards.

Spinal Stretch

1 As you tilt from your hips to lower your upper body, the passive partner sinks her back down onto yours, allowing her head and neck to relax backwards. Check that she is feeling safe before you lift her upwards.

Lower Your Torso

2 Begin to lower your torso to lift your partner's feet away from the ground so the full weight of her back is released towards your body. It is important for her shoulders and neck to remain relaxed. Move very slowly and in tune with her. Stay balanced and secure on your own feet and legs, and breathe easily, taking care to remain relaxed in your own body.

Lifting Off

3 As you lift her higher off the ground, her spine receives a good slow stretch. She should breathe fully into her chest and abdomen. Remain in this position for some moments, and then slowly put her back down, by extending gently upwards from your hips. Her feet need firm contact with the floor before you straighten up.

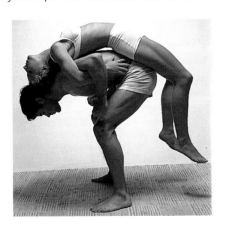

Contrasting Physiques

▶ It is possible for two people of different sizes to do this exercise provided you maintain stability and relaxation. However, common sense will guide you as to whether the weight or height differences are too great to attempt it. The first priority is to ensure that there is no danger of you straining your back or spine in any exercise.

Contraception

Contraception is an important consideration for most sexually active people, as a way of avoiding unwanted pregnancy or as an aid to family planning. It is important to keep in mind, however, that no method is 100 per cent reliable, and some forms of contraception do not protect against HIV or other sexually transmitted diseases. Condoms have been shown to be effective against these risks and to play an invaluable role in safer sex, as well as guarding against conception.

There is now a much wider choice of contraceptive methods than ever before, and most are readily available. The various forms are discussed below, and their suitability for you can best be determined by consulting a health practitioner. Changing lifestyles or needs, or relevant health issues, may require that you re-evaluate the type of contraceptive you are currently using. This is easily done in consultation with your doctor or local family planning clinic.

It is important, as a sexually active person, to take a responsible attitude to contraception and to avoid spreading sexually transmitted diseases. Some forms of contraception carry health risks, which you should take into account when choosing the most suitable method for you, bearing in mind factors such as your medical condition, weight, age and lifestyle.

However, it is worth bearing in mind that pregnancy and childbirth also involve slight risks, to say nothing of the distress of an unwanted pregnancy. The various methods now available should make the decision on these matters easier and ensure your choice is best suited to the specific needs of you and your partner.

The failure rates quoted in this section are based on the theoretical number of pregnancies that can be expected within one year among 100 couples having regular sex and using the particular form of contraception mentioned. The risk of failure is obviously increased if a contraceptive method is used incorrectly.

HORMONAL METHODS

Oral Contraceptive Pill

The oral contraceptive pill has been used by millions of women since its introduction in the early 1960s. There are currently over 60 million women world-wide using this method. If used correctly, the pill is a highly reliable form of contraception – up to 99 per cent effective. The advantage of the pill is that couples do not have to think about contraception (so long as it is taken on the days and at the times specified) and so it does not interfere with their spontaneity.

The pill works by suppressing normal control of a woman's sex hormone system, thereby artificially regulating her menstrual cycle. Most forms of the pill contain a combination of progestogen and synthetic oestrogen, which mimic the female hormones progesterone and oestrogen. The effect is to prevent ovulation, make the cervical mucus impenetrable to sperm, and alter the lining of the uterus so that a fertilized egg cannot implant in it.

The combined pill is taken on 21 days out of 28 – with seven pill-free days. It is available in three forms: monophasic, biphasic and triphasic. Monophasic pills release constant doses of hormones. Biphasic and triphasic pills release staged doses – in two phases and three phases respectively – to mimic the normal pattern of female hormone production more closely.

The combined pill may be less effective if it is taken more than 12 hours late, or if there is any vomiting or diarrhoea. Other medications, such as antibiotics, sedatives and some painkillers, may also alter the efficacy of the combined pill. In any of these cases, an additional form of contraception should be used until the end of the cycle.

Studies have linked the combined pill with an increased risk of cardio-vascular disease, and liver and cervical cancer, but it seems to offer protection against ovarian cancer, cancer of the endometrium (the lining of the uterus), ovarian cysts, non-cancerous breast tumours, fibroids, and ectopic pregnancy. Medical opinion is divided on the link between hormonal pills and breast cancer.

All women who use hormonal contraceptive methods should have regular breast examinations, cervical smears, and six-monthly check-ups of blood pressure and weight.

The combined pill does have some serious side-effects such as increased risk of blood clots in the arteries and veins. This risk is much greater in women over the age of 35, smokers, and those who are very overweight. It is not usually prescribed for women in these high-risk categories. Some of the other side-effects of the pill reported include breast tenderness, mood swings, weight gain, water retention, and loss of libido. Vaginal infections, such as thrush, are also more common among contraceptive pill users.

Mini-Pill

Another form of hormonal contraception is the progestogen-only pill, or mini-pill, which is taken every day, without a break. It uses only very low doses of progestogen, so it must be taken at the same time each day to prevent fertilization, and never more than three hours late. It has fewer side-effects than the combined pill but there is a higher failure rate (up to four per cent).

Because it does not contain oestrogen, which is the hormone that has been linked to thrombosis, or blood clots forming in the veins and arteries, it may be a better alternative in certain cases. It is associated with a higher risk of breast cancer than the combined pill, particularly among women who have taken the drug for over five years. Some women who use it may have irregular periods, or light spotting between periods.

Implants

Implants are another hormonal method of birth control. Six tiny, flexible capsules are inserted under the skin of the upper arm. This requires minor surgery, which is carried out under a local anaesthetic. Once in place, the capsules release low levels of progestogen directly into the bloodstream. Implants rarely cause discomfort, and they provide contraceptive protection for up to five years. They may cause changes in menstruation, producing either heavier periods or irregular periods, and weight gain. They also require minor surgery to be taken out.

Fertility is restored soon after removal of the implants. As this method does not contain oestrogen, it may be suitable for women who cannot use the combined pill.

Injectable Contraceptives

In this method, an injection of progestogen is given in a muscle during the first five days of menstruation. It provides contraceptive protection for eight to twelve weeks. Though its effectiveness rivals that of the pill, it is mostly prescribed in exceptional circumstances. These include women who have just been immunized against rubella, when pregnancy could result in birth defects in the foetus; women whose partners have recently had a vasectomy, until tests can show there are no longer sperm present; and women who are unable to use other forms of birth control. Once injected the contraceptive action cannot be reversed and there may also be a delay before fertility returns. Menstrual disturbances, weight gain and a delay in fertility are the most common side-effects.

BARRIER METHODS

IUD

The IUD (intra-uterine device, or "coil") is a T-shaped appliance that is inserted through the cervix into the uterus. It is not known exactly how the IUD works. It was previously thought that it prevents a fertilized ovum implanting in the lining of the uterus, but research now suggests its main action is to make conditions in the uterus hostile to sperm.

Many IUDs are made of plastic, or copper wire on a plastic frame. Some have a silver core and there are versions that also release progestogen. IUDs have two nylon threads that hang down into the vagina, enabling the woman to check each month whether the device is still in place. Some forms must be replaced every two to three years, others can be left in the womb for up to five years, and some last over ten years. Regular check-ups will be necessary.

An IUD should only be inserted by a doctor. This is usually done during menstruation because the cervix is slightly dilated at this time, and there is little likelihood that the woman is pregnant. An IUD can, however, be expelled from the uterus soon after insertion or in the first three months. Sometimes, though rarely, the IUD can dislodge and perforate the wall of the uterus. Usually, this is signalled by sharp pains in the lower abdomen and vaginal bleeding. Many users experience heavier, more painful periods, especially in the first few months. It also makes a woman's reproductive system more vulnerable to infections such as PID (pelvic inflammatory disease) which, when untreated, can lead to infertility. It is therefore not advised for younger women, or those who have had no children, or women with a history of sexually transmitted diseases.

The IUD is a very effective form of birth control with a protection rate similar to the combined pill. However, if pregnancy does occur with an IUD in place there is a higher risk of miscarriage, either if it is left in place or at the time of removal. It does not protect against STDs and is better suited to women in monogamous relationships.

Spermicides

Spermicides are available in many different forms, most often as vaginal creams, gels, foams, pessaries and tablets. A contraceptive film is also available, which is packed between squares of silver foil for easy handling. Spermicides are available from the chemist without a prescription and most contain the active ingredient Nonoxynol-9. They usually offer protection for only one episode of intercourse, and must be re-applied before sex is repeated. On their own, they are not highly effective as a contraceptive, with failure rates as high as 25 per cent.

Spermicides are most effective when used in conjunction with another barrier method, such as the condom, diaphragm, cap or sponge (see below). They may cause minor irritations or allergies in either partner. Some spermicides may damage condoms and diaphragms, so only recommended types should be used. Recent tests show that Nonoxynol-9 can kill the HIV virus, the disease responsible for AIDS.

The Diaphragm

The diaphragm is a soft rubber dome, reinforced with a flexible metal spring in the rim, that is placed inside the vagina so that it covers the cervix. It is easily fitted by the user herself, simply by pressing two sides together so it can be inserted. When used consistently with spermicide, placed on the surfaces of the diaphragm before insertion, it can provide a very safe form of birth control – up to 98 per cent effective – and does not interfere with a woman's hormonal balance. However, when used without spermicide, the failure rate can be as high as 15 per cent. The diaphragm must be left in place for at least six hours after sexual intercourse, but no longer than 24 hours. Additional spermicide must be applied before intercourse is repeated.

As the diaphragm is made of a relatively thin form of rubber, it must be checked for signs of deterioration, such as small cuts or tears, before each use. It should also be checked for size every six months as childbirth, miscarriage, or weight gain or loss of more than 3kg/7lb in the user can make it less effective. In such a case a more appropriate size should be fitted. Some women find it difficult to insert, though with practice it usually becomes easier. It can also impair spontaneity for it needs to be inserted before lovemaking. Some women cope with this by inserting it earlier in the evening, but they should keep in mind that spermicide loses a great deal of its potency after three hours and more should be added prior to intercourse.

The diaphragm puts pressure on the bladder and so is not recommended for women who suffer from recurrent cystitis or other urinary infections. A few women are allergic to the rubber of the diaphragm and will not be able to tolerate it. There is a risk of toxic shock syndrome if the diaphragm is worn continuously, especially during a period.

The Cap

The cap functions very much like the diaphragm but is smaller, fitting snugly over the cervix where it is held in place by suction. It has the same success rate as the diaphragm and must be used in conjunction with spermicide to be most effective. It must also be left in place for six hours after sexual intercourse. Additional spermicide should be inserted if sexual intercourse is repeated. Like the diaphragm, its main drawback is that it may detract from spontaneity as it needs to be fitted prior to intercourse.

The Condom

The condom is one of the oldest forms of contraception. Condoms are enjoying renewed popularity for their ability to provide protection against HIV and other sexually transmitted diseases. They are made of fine latex rubber with a teat at the end to collect sperm. To provide maximum protection, the condom should be fitted prior to any genital contact. The condom should be rolled down evenly over the erect penis, taking care to expel all the air from the tip. After ejaculation, the man should withdraw his penis, holding the base of the condom so that no sperm escapes into the vagina.

Only water-based lubricants should be used; oil-based products can cause the rubber to deteriorate. Most condoms contain spermicide and this usually provides sufficient lubrication. Condoms should always be handled with care and checked for signs of damage or ageing. They should not be carried in pockets or wallets where they can get damaged.

Some men complain of a loss of sensation when using condoms, but this is less of a problem nowadays as modern condoms are made of a very thin form of latex. Indeed, any reduced sensitivity may be an advantage for men who suffer premature ejaculation, or who wish to extend lovemaking. Fitting a condom can become part of foreplay so it does not detract from the spontaneity.

Apart from a very small number who are allergic to rubber, there is nothing to prevent most people from using them. Condoms play an invaluable role in safer sex. Their use is particularly recommended with new or casual partners. Used consistently, they are up to 98 per cent effective.

The Female Condom

The female condom, which was developed by a Danish physician in the 1980s, is an innovation in birth control. Like the male condom, it has the added benefit of protecting the user against sexually transmitted diseases, including HIV.

The female condom is a long, loose tube, about 17.5 cm/7in in length, which is closed at one end. It has a smaller fixed ring which is inserted into the vagina and pushed in as far as possible to cover the cervix. A larger ring remains outside and is pushed back against the labia during intercourse. The female condom is pre-lubricated, and made of flexible polyurethane, which is thinner than latex, so there is not so much loss of sensitivity. It is also very loose so it does not have the same constricting feeling as its male counterpart, but is likely to affect sensation nevertheless.

Some women find it rather uncomfortable, but it has the advantage of not requiring the man to withdraw immediately, as is the case with the male condom. Polyurethane is also stronger and more durable than latex, so is less likely to break during intercourse. As it is heavily lubricated, the female condom may be of benefit to women following childbirth or suffering vaginal dryness, around the time of the menopause, for example. Some trials claim a success rate similar to the male condom, though other studies suggest it may be less effective, with failure rates of up to 25 per cent.

The Sponge

The sponge is made of soft polythene foam, impregnated with Nonoxynol-9 spermicide. In order to activate the spermicide, the sponge should be moistened with water before insertion. It is placed as far into the vagina as it will go, and should cover the cervix. It can be inserted any time before sex and must be removed no longer than 30 hours afterwards (but must be left in for at least six hours).

The spermicide component kills sperm for up to 48 hours, regardless of the number of times intercourse takes place. Its major disadvantage is that it has a high failure rate, up to 25 per cent, and should be used with a condom to protect against the risk of pregnancy. A small number of women, between three and five per cent, are allergic to the spermicide.

POST-COITAL CONTRACEPTION

The "Morning-After" Pill

If a woman has had unprotected sexual intercourse, or suspects her method of contraception has failed and is concerned about pregnancy, she can obtain the morning-after pill from her doctor. This emergency contraception is a form of hormonal pill which is taken in double doses – that is, two pills at a time. The first dose is taken within 72 hours of intercourse, and the second dose 12 hours later. Many users experience nausea and breast tenderness.

If vomiting occurs, another dose will be necessary as the pills may not have been absorbed by the body. It does not seem to have any other adverse effects, though it may be unsuitable for women who have been advised not to use other forms of hormonal contraception. Should the morning-after pill fail, it is not yet known what effects there may be on the developing foetus.

Post-Coital IUD

The IUD can also be used as a method of emergency contraception, and has the advantage that it can be used up to five days after unprotected sex, or within five days after the release of an egg. It is not recommended for women who have not had children, or where there is a risk of sexually transmitted disease, for example in cases of rape. As a method of post-coital contraception the IUD is credited with a 100 per cent success rate, to date.

STERILIZATION

Sterilization is a permanent form of birth control, and though it may be reversed, there is no guarantee that fertility will be restored. It is an option that is favoured by people who already have children. It is usually inadvisable in young people, or those who have not had children, for if they have a change of heart later, reversal may not be successful. Counselling is advisable prior to deciding on sterilization.

Vasectomy

A vasectomy is a relatively minor surgical procedure that is usually carried out under local anaesthetic, taking around ten to 15 minutes. It involves cutting and tying back the vasa deferentia, the tubes which carry sperm from the testicles. Most men will need one or two days to recover fully from the operation.

The man's semen may still contain active sperm between six to eight weeks after a vasectomy, so it is important that an alternative means of birth control is used during this time until two separate semen samples have been examined and shown to be free of sperm.

Quick Guide to Contraception

METHOD: **The Combined Pill**

Risks:

✘ Side-effects: mood swings, nausea, weight gain, loss of libido, headaches

✘ Increased risk of blood clots, especially in the overweight and smokers aged over 35

✘ Possible increased risk of cardiovascular disease, and liver, breast and cervical cancer

Benefits:

✔ Highly effective as a contraceptive

✔ Protection against cancer of the ovaries and endometrium

✔ Lighter periods

✔ Reduced risk of ovarian cysts

METHOD: **The Mini-Pill**

Risks:

✘ Small increased risk of ovarian cysts

✘ Less effective than the combined pill

✘ Possible increased risk of breast cancer

Benefits:

✔ Possible protection against ovarian cancer

✔ Side-effects are less severe than the combined pill

METHOD: **Hormonal Implants**

Risks:

✘ Complications have been reported in some women during insertion or removal of implants

✘ Heavy, irregular or absent periods

✘ Weight gain

Benefits:

✔ Does not interrupt spontaneity of sexual intercourse

✔ Provides effective contraception for up to five years or until removed

METHOD: **Hormonal Injection**

Risks:

✘ Heavy, irregular or absent periods

✘ Weight gain

✘ Delay in return of fertility

Benefits:

✔ Reduced risk of ovarian and endometrial cancer

✔ Reduced risk of ovarian cysts

✔ Does not interrupt spontaneity of sexual intercourse

METHOD: **IUD**

Risks:

✘ Increased risk of PID and other pelvic infections

✘ Increased risk of ectopic pregnancy

✘ Heavier periods in many users

Benefits:

✔ Very effective form of birth control

✔ Can be removed without delay in return of fertility

METHOD: **Diaphragm/Cap**

Risks:

✘ Slight risk of toxic shock syndrome

✘ Can interrupt spontaneity of sexual intercourse

✘ Not as effective without the use of a spermicide

Benefits:

✔ Does not interfere with a woman's hormonal balance

✔ Some protection against genital warts

✔ Some protection against cervical cancer

✔ Some protection against HIV and other sexually transmitted diseases, particularly when used with spermicide

METHOD: **Condom**

Risks:

✘ It may break or tear during intercourse

✘ Can interrupt spontaneity of sexual intercourse

Benefits:

✔ Protects against HIV and other sexually transmitted diseases

METHOD: **The Sponge**

Risks:

✘ Relatively high failure rate

Benefits:

✔ Once in place it can be left for 24 hours

METHOD: **Vasectomy**

Risks:

✘ Psychological regret about loss of fertility

✘ Must generally be considered irreversible

Benefits:

✔ Freedom from fear of impregnating partner

METHOD: **Female Sterilization**

Risks:

✘ Psychological regret about loss of fertility

✘ Must generally be considered irreversible

✘ Some women experience heavier periods

Benefits:

✔ Freedom from fear of pregnancy

METHOD: **Natural Family Planning**

Risks:

✘ Without adequate tuition, motivation and commitment, this is an unreliable form of birth control

Benefits:

✔ Morally acceptable for couples that don't want to use artificial means of contraception

✔ Gives better insight of how a woman's body functions

METHOD: **Coitus Interruptus**

Risks:

✘ Too unreliable

On rare occasions, the ends of a vas deferens may rejoin spontaneously, but usually a vasectomy is a highly effective form of birth control. Reversal techniques using micro-surgery are becoming increasingly successful, but there is always the risk that anti-sperm antibodies will have been produced that will render the man infertile. Vasectomy should therefore be considered irreversible and only contemplated if the man is sure he has completed his family.

Female Sterilization

Female sterilization is growing in popularity, particularly among those women who have had children. It is a more complicated operation than a vasectomy, and as it is usually carried out under general anaesthetic carries a greater risk. It involves blocking the Fallopian tubes, which carry eggs from the ovaries to the uterus, by cutting, cauterizing or attaching clips to them. This is normally done via a small incision made in the lower abdomen just above the pubic bone.

Sterilization does not usually require an overnight stay in the hospital and its effect is immediate. There may be some pain for a couple of days, while gas pumped into the abdomen during the operation gradually disperses. For many women who have had children, sterilization removes the fear of pregnancy. It is not recommended in younger women or those that have had no children. Some women do experience heavier periods after sterilization. Reversal is a costly and difficult process, and not always effective, though there is a 40 to 80 per cent chance of success. Like male sterilization, it should only be considered if a woman is sure she has completed her family.

NATURAL FAMILY PLANNING (THE RHYTHM METHOD)

Once an egg has been released at ovulation it can only survive for around 24 hours. Sperm have a longer life span, but conditions must be suitable for them. About six days before ovulation, the cervix starts producing a special kind of mucus that provides just the right kind of environment for the sperm. They cannot live long without it, but when it is present they can survive for up to five days, lying in wait ready to fertilize the egg as soon as it is released. Natural family planning is about learning to recognize the changes in a woman's body that indicate her fertile time. Then, unless the couple plan to have a baby, they can abstain from sex during those days or use a barrier method of contraception.

It may be the only option for couples who, for moral or religious reasons, choose not to use artificial means of birth control. It can also be used by women who want to feel they are in tune with their bodies, or who do not find other methods of birth control satisfactory, or who are actively trying to get pregnant.

There are various forms of natural family planning. The most widely practised is the sympto-thermal method, which uses a combination of factors to recognize the fertile stage. These include changes in basal body temperature (her temperature at rest, usually taken soon after waking in the morning), changes in cervical mucus, and changes in the softness, firmness and position of the cervix. Other signs include pain or discomfort in the back, lower abdomen, or breasts. Such changes need to be recorded on a chart, and a woman will usually have to monitor these symptoms and signs over several cycles before she begins to recognize a pattern.

For example, following ovulation a woman's basal body temperature rises by a very small amount and stays at this level until the onset of her next period. This slight change can only be detected by a special fertility thermometer, available from chemists and family planning clinics. Her mucus also alters, from scant, sticky, white or absent, often becoming more profuse, and usually changing to a slippery and stretchy texture that may be clear or slightly cloudy. Some women also experience pain or discomfort at the time of ovulation. Careful monitoring of these various signs should pinpoint the fertile days.

Natural family planning is a complicated procedure that requires motivation, commitment and careful observation of the rules. Women need to learn the correct method from a properly trained natural family planning teacher before they use it as their only form of birth control. When practised conscientiously it has a 97 per cent success rate, which compares with the IUD and hormonal contraception.

COITUS INTERRUPTUS/ WITHDRAWAL

Coitus interruptus, also known as the withdrawal method, is probably the most widely used form of birth control in the world and also the most unreliable. It involves withdrawing the penis from the vagina just prior to ejaculation. As a man's pre-ejaculatory fluid can contain millions of sperm, and accidents are unavoidable, this method has a very high failure rate.

STDs *(Sexually Transmitted Diseases)*

Sexually transmitted diseases (STDs) can have unpleasant and often serious consequences. The world-wide spread of AIDS, a potentially fatal condition arising from a sexually transmitted disease, has highlighted more than ever the need to avoid high-risk sexual practices. If you suspect that you have caught a sexually transmitted disease, it is vital that you seek medical attention at the first opportunity. With all STDs, the infected person should inform all known sexual partners so that they too can be examined and receive the appropriate treatment.

Never ignore the symptoms of a sexually transmitted disease. Most STDs respond well to prompt treatment but delay can allow the disease to spread and risks infertility, crippling side-effects and even death. Medical aid is available from your doctor or, if you prefer, at an STD or GUM (genito-urinary medicine) clinic, where medical staff have specialist knowledge. At such clinics, treatment is confidential and visitors can remain anonymous, if they wish. They will, however, be asked for the names of sexual partners who may be at risk, as the clinic will need to get in touch with them to arrange treatment. They will be contacted in strict confidence. Below, in alphabetical order, are listed the most common sexually transmitted diseases.

Candidiasis (Thrush)

Candidiasis, or thrush, is a common complaint. It is caused by a yeast-like fungus called *Candida albicans* that lives, usually quite harmlessly, in the mouth, intestinal tract and vagina. It is normally kept under control by bacteria that also live in these locations. A warm, moist environment is needed for the fungus to thrive, so the vagina makes an ideal home.

Anything that alters conditions in the vagina can tip the balance in favour of the fungus and enable it to multiply. Tight and confining clothing, illness, or antibiotics, which can destroy the beneficial bacteria, may trigger an outbreak. It is more common in pregnant women, diabetics, and those using hormonal contraceptives. Thrush can also be contracted through sex, and every year thousands of people with the condition visit STD clinics.

Symptoms vary. In women, there may be intense itching of the vulva, with soreness, redness and swelling around the vagina, vulva or anus. They may experience a burning sensation during sex, and when urinating, and some may notice a thick, white, yeast-smelling discharge, which has the consistency of cottage cheese. Not all women show this symptom, however.

In men, a rash may appear on the penis and can occasionally spread to the scrotum. Some may notice a slight burning sensation on the penis during or after sexual intercourse. Thrush can cause considerable discomfort, particularly in those who are prone to recurrences.

The condition is usually treated with antifungal drugs, often as creams or pessaries. The partner should be treated at the same time to prevent re-infection. Other measures may be needed such as wearing loose, natural clothing, and sterilizing underwear and towels. Women who use hormonal contraceptives may be advised to use an alternative form of birth control.

Chancroid

Chancroid is a sexually transmitted disease caused by the bacterium *Haemophylus ducreyi*. It is most often found in tropical countries, mainly through contact with prostitutes, but is becoming more common in the West because of increased international travel. There is an incubation period of up to one week before a painful ulcer forms on the penis or near the entrance to the vagina. There may also be a painful swelling in the groin. If the disease is not treated, abscesses can form in the groin which leave deep scars. Chancroid is usually treated with an antibiotic such as erythromycin.

Chlamydia

Chlamydia trachomatis, a microorganism similar to a bacterium, is the most prevalent STD in the West. It is one of the main causes of a disorder called non-specific urethritis, or NSU (see below) which can lead to infertility. Chlamydia can be transmitted by vaginal, anal, or oral sex, or it can be passed on to a baby during childbirth.

Men may experience a burning sensation when urinating, a whitish discharge from the urethra, and pain and swelling of the testicles, but often there are no symptoms. In women, symptoms are even less common but some may notice pain or a burning sensation when urinating, or a cloudy, white discharge.

If chlamydia remains undetected it can spread through the reproductive tract resulting in a potentially life-threatening condition called pelvic inflammatory disease (PID), itself a major cause of infertility. Chlamydia is treated with antibiotics such as tetracycline and erythromycin. Partners should be treated at the same time, to avoid re-infection.

Genital Herpes

Genital herpes is caused by the *Herpes simplex* virus, which produces painful blisters on or near the genitals. *Herpes simplex* occurs in two main forms. The first, type I, causes cold sores. It is type II that causes genital herpes. The latter form is usually transmitted by sexual contact, including oral sex, and can enter the body through the mucous membranes, or through tiny tears in the skin. It is very infectious and the risk of catching the disease greatly increases if an individual has multiple sexual partners.

There is an incubation period of three to six days, followed by the appearance of a group of small, painful blisters on or near the genitals. These blisters break open and then heal, over a period of 10 to 20 days. The initial attack of genital herpes is usually accompanied by symptoms such as fever, headaches, muscular pain and itching. Further outbreaks will usually cause a recurrence of the blisters.

Once a person has become infected the virus is with them for life, although up to 20 per cent only have one attack. For the rest, the flare-ups usually grow steadily less intense over time. Various factors can cause outbreaks, including stress, anxiety, depression, or illness. Some people are able to anticipate an attack, two or three days beforehand, when they notice symptoms such as tingling, itching, or burning sensa-

tions in the genitals. Sexual contact should be avoided during and just before an outbreak, as the condition is highly infectious at this time. There is no cure for genital herpes, but anti-viral drugs such as acyclovir can reduce the pain and speed up healing. Genital herpes may play a part in cervical cancer, so infected women should be sure to have annual cervical smear tests.

Genital Warts

Genital warts are caused by the human *papillomavirus,* which is sexually transmitted. The warts are soft and dry, and greyish-pink in colour. Usually painless, they are found on or near the genitals and anus. There is an incubation period of six to eight weeks after exposure. The virus is transmitted by direct contact with the warts, although the virus has also been found in semen. Like genital herpes, genital warts have been linked with cervical cancer, so yearly cervical smears are advisable for affected women.

Genital warts may be destroyed by caustic chemicals, such as podophyllin, or by laser surgery, or liquid nitrogen. As the virus remains in the tissues, however, genital warts tend to recur. Even when warts are not present, affected people should use condoms to avoid transmitting the virus to partners.

Gonorrhoea ("The Clap")

Gonorrhoea is an infection caused by the bacterium *Neisseria gonorrhoea.* It is one of the most common sexually transmitted diseases and is found principally among teenagers and young adults who have several sexual partners. It can be passed on during vaginal, anal, or oral sex, and an

infected woman can transmit the disease to her baby during childbirth. Men are more likely than women to show symptoms. They may experience soreness or swelling at the tip of the penis, and a burning sensation when passing urine, often accompanied by a milky discharge from the urethra, two to ten days after infection. The discharge may become thicker, and yellowish in colour, and sometimes contains traces of blood.

Up to 60 per cent of infected women have mild symptoms, or none at all. They may urinate more often, and urination may be painful. There may be a watery, yellow or greenish discharge from the urethra. If the cervix has been infected, there may be vaginal discharge and abnormal menstrual bleeding.

Gonorrhoea is a common cause of infertility and can lead to pelvic inflammatory disease (PID). In a few cases, the infection can spread through the bloodstream, causing conditions as diverse as arthritis, skin rashes, and septicaemia, and even leading to brain damage and death, in severe cases. The disease is easily treated with penicillin antibiotics (or suitable alternatives, for those allergic to such drugs) and, as with all STDs, sexual partners must be contacted so they can receive treatment as well.

Hepatitis

Hepatitis is a serious and potentially fatal disease in which the liver becomes badly inflamed, leading to serious tissue damage. It can be caused by alcohol abuse, drugs, poisons, chemicals, and certain viruses. Of the different forms of viral hepatitis, the two most common are hepatitis A and B. Type A is usually caught from contaminated food or water. Hepatitis B is mainly passed on during sex, or via contaminated needles, particularly among drug users.

It has an incubation period of a few weeks to several months. Sufferers may have a flu-like illness, with nausea and vomiting, followed by jaundice. Some carriers, however, show no symptoms and yet are still be able to infect others. Up to ten per cent of sufferers go on to develop the chronic, or long-term, form of the disease resulting in steadily increasing liver damage.

There is no specific treatment, other than bed rest, a good diet, and anti-inflammatory drugs. However, there is a vaccine against hepatitis B which is recommended for anyone at particular risk, including those with multiple sexual partners (homosexual or heterosexual), intravenous drug users, health care workers, and relatives of carriers.

HIV/AIDS

HIV (human immunodeficiency virus) is a disease that is most often transmitted through unprotected sexual intercourse and by sharing needles and syringes among intravenous drug users. HIV can attack the brain directly, but most often it targets white blood cells called T-4 cells, which are vital to the body's immune system.

Over a period of time, the immune system is so badly impaired that the body becomes vulnerable to a range of opportunistic infections and cancers. This latter, potentially fatal, stage is called AIDS (acquired immune deficiency syndrome). Some of these illnesses, such as Karposi's sarcoma or Pneumocystis carinii, are rare or relatively harmless among non-AIDS sufferers, but life-threatening in those with impaired immune systems.

The rate at which HIV progresses to AIDS is highly variable. Some people develop AIDS within months, while others have milder symptoms for years, a condition known as ARC (AIDS-related complex). They may have periods of good health, interspersed with periods of illness. Some infected people show no symptoms and yet are capable of infecting others. It can take up to ten years or more for the symptoms of full-blown AIDS to develop.

HIV is easily killed outside the body and there is no known risk through ordinary social contact, such as hugging, sharing a meal, or using another person's cups, cutlery, or crockery. The main risk is through the exchange of body fluids. This is why HIV can be passed on through all forms of penetrative sex, especially if there are cuts, tears, or sores in the vagina or anus, or on the penis or cervix.

There is a greater risk if a person has already contracted genital herpes or warts. While HIV is present in all body fluids of an infected person, particularly in semen, vaginal fluids and blood, the risk of transmission in saliva is considered to be minimal. Mothers can transmit HIV to their babies, at birth or through breast-feeding. In the past, HIV has been contracted through contaminated blood and blood products, but this risk is now negligible in the West, with the introduction of screening and heat treatment of donor blood. Health workers can be at risk through accidental injury with a contaminated needle.

Those who suspect they may have HIV, especially people in high-risk categories, can have a blood test to determine whether they have been infected. This test detects whether the body has developed antibodies to try to fight the disease. Those found to have developed antibodies are said to be HIV-positive. A negative result means either that individuals do not have the virus, or that their body has not yet made antibodies, which take two to three months to develop. If you're considering having an HIV test it is vital that you first get specialist counselling to help you understand the implications if the result is positive.

At present there is no vaccine against HIV and no cure for HIV or AIDS, though symptoms and complications can often be treated with antibiotics, anti-cancer drugs and radiotherapy. Anti-viral drugs such as AZT (zidovudine) and acyclovir may reduce the speed at which AIDS develops.

To reduce the risk of HIV infection, individuals should practise safer sex if they are unsure of a partner's sexual history. This means finding safer alternatives to penetrative sex, such as mutual masturbation, or using condoms or other forms of latex barrier. This applies both to casual sex, and sex with long-term partners who might previously have been at risk of acquiring HIV. Intravenous drug users should never share needles and syringes.

NSU

NSU (or non-specific urethritis) is inflammation of the urethra, the tube through which urine passes out of the body, due to causes other than gonorrhoea. It is a fairly common complaint. The main symptom is pain when urinating, which is sometimes, but not always, accompanied by a discharge. There can be over 70 causes of NSU, the most common being chlamydia (see previous page) and trichomonas (see below) infection. It is usually sexually transmitted.

Treatment can be difficult unless the disease responsible is identified. This is usually done by taking samples from the opening of the urethra, or by examining a urine sample (usually taken in the morning when there is the highest buildup of organisms). The choice of medication depends on the underlying cause, although it is most likely to be cured by antibiotics. Partners of those with NSU should also be treated to avoid re-infection.

Pubic Lice ("Crabs")

Pubic lice, *Phthiris pubis*, are a parasitic form of insect. They are more commonly known as crabs because of the crab-like claws by which they attach themselves to hairs. They are most likely to infest the pubic region, but they can be found on all body hairs – even the eyebrows. They do not usually infest the scalp.

Crabs are mainly spread by sexual contact, though they can also be caught from infested bedding or clothing, or from lavatory seats. The eggs are laid at the base of the pubic hairs and hatch about a week later. Pubic lice puncture the skin to feed on blood, which causes the intense itching and irritation. Treatment is with insecticide lotion, available on prescription or from the pharmacist, applied to infected areas. Partners should also be treated to avoid re-infection, and clothes and bedding should be washed in very hot water.

Syphilis

Syphilis, a sexually transmitted disease caused by the bacterium *Treponema pallidum*, was introduced into Europe from North America during the late 15th century. It soon reached epidemic proportions, causing many deaths. Syphilis continued to spread in the following centuries, although its virulence abated. The discovery of penicillin in the 1940s brought it under control.

The bacterium enters the body via broken skin or the mucous membranes, in and around the mouth, genitals and anus. It is highly contagious and can be passed on by any intimate contact, including penetrative sex, oral sex, and even kissing. Unlike with most other STDs, condoms do not give total protection against syphilis.

The disease has four stages: primary, secondary, latent and tertiary. During the primary stage, the first symptoms of syphilis appear after an incubation period of just under a month. A small, painless ulcer will appear at the site of transmission, usually around the genitals or anus, but sometimes the lips, throat or fingers. This ulcer usually disappears after six weeks.

The secondary stage usually occurs up to three months after initial infection. It is marked by a variety of symptoms, the most common being a skin rash, but there may be fever, headaches, sore throat, swollen lymph nodes, aches and pains, loss of hair, and pink patches may appear on the skin. In some cases, there may be meningitis (inflammation of the membranes surrounding the brain), eye infection, or kidney problems.

If untreated, the sufferer enters the latent period, when symptoms may lie dormant for twenty years or more. Symptoms may recur in some sufferers. The tertiary phase is very serious and usually involves destruction of tissues and internal organs, such as damage to the heart, blood vessels, nervous system, and brain, resulting in heart disease, mental disorders, paralysis, and death.

Syphilis is usually identified with a blood test. The disease can be tackled effectively with penicillin or other antibiotics, although 50 per cent of infected people suffer a severe reaction to treatment as the body responds to the death of large numbers of bacteria.

Trichomoniasis

Trichomoniasis (TV) is an infection caused by a single-celled parasite, or protozoon, called *Trichomonas vaginalis*. This highly infectious micro-organism is a common cause of vaginitis, or inflammation of the vagina, and is almost exclusively transmitted sexually.

Symptoms, if any, start between four days and three weeks after sexual contact and can show as a thin vaginal discharge that is yellow or green, and frothy, and usually has an offensive smell. In addition, some women may experience vaginal pain and itching, especially during sexual intercourse. These symptoms usually worsen during or after menstruation. Many women, however, suffer no symptoms at all.

Men don't usually show symptoms, although a few may notice a slight discharge and find urinating painful. The condition usually responds to treatment with the antiprotozoal drug metronidazole. The sexual partner should also be treated to avoid re-infection.